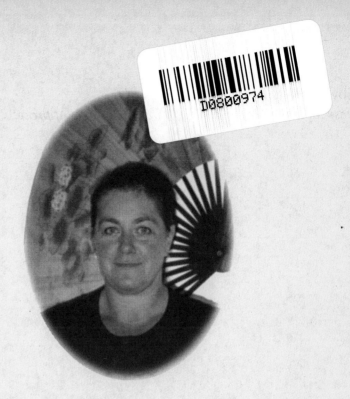

Bronwyn Whitlocke is a practising Shiatsu therapist and Traditional Chinese Medicine herbalist-acupuncturist. She believes we can achieve good health if we use natural and non-intrusive remedies. She takes a commonsense approach to encouraging us to understand and maintain our own health.

Also by Bronwyn Whitlocke
Chinese Medicine for Women: A Common Sense Approach

SHIATSU THERAPY FOR PREGNANCY

A HANDBOOK FOR THE THERAPIST
AND SUPPORT PERSON

BRONWYN WHITLOCKE

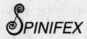

Spinifex Press Pty Ltd
504 Queensberry Street
North Melbourne, Victoria 3051
Australia
women@spinifexpress.com.au
http://www.spinifexpress.com.au

Edited by Deborah Doyle (Living Proof – Book Editing)
Indexed by Max McMaster
Cover designed by Deb Snibson (Modern Art Production Group)
Illustrated by Sonia Kretschmar
Text designed and typeset by Claire Warren
Made and printed in Australia by Australian Print Group

National Library of Australia
Cataloguing-in-Publication data:

Whitlocke, Bronwyn, 1951–
    Shiatsu therapy for pregnancy: a handbook for the therapist and support person.
    Bibliography.
    Includes index.
    ISBN 1 875559 81 7

    1. Prenatal care. 2. Acupressure. 3. Pregnancy. 4. Postnatal care. I. Title.
618.24

I dedicate the book to my daughter Jessica
for her unfailing love and support.

Author's note

In this book, the illustrations of meridians and points are intended to be a guide only.

I wish to thank Jessica Watson and Liz Carlyon for agreeing to model for the photographs, Phillip Lamb for helping with the photography, and Joanne Hafey and Patricia Sharp for providing support and comments when I was writing the book.

Contents

Introduction

I have written this book in order to help the therapist establish relevant treatments for women's antenatal and postnatal care. I also intend the book to be used by the recipient's support person, for whom I have included separate, easily identifiable sections headed "A suggested treatment for the support person to apply". Throughout the book, I refer to both the pregnant woman and the new mother as the *recipient* of the Shiatsu therapy.

I discuss common conditions and issues that are relevant to the recipient. Some pressure points – which I refer to simply as *points* – are contraindicated in pregnancy, so I repeat them in each treatment section. If you wish to find out more about the concepts of Traditional Chinese Medicine, please refer to my book *Chinese Medicine for Women: A Common Sense Approach*, published by Spinifex Press in 1997: I intend it to be this book's companion.

In this book, I discuss simple Shiatsu techniques for the support person to apply to the woman, techniques for the woman to apply to herself, and more-involved techniques for the therapist to apply to the woman. For conditions specifically related to pregnancy, I list the specific Shiatsu points separately for both the therapist and the support person. I do this because some points are powerful movers of Qi, and a qualified therapist knows how to use them without causing the recipient harm.

I recommend that the support person who is new to Shiatsu use only the points that are listed for him or her to use.

The support person might not obtain the results the therapist obtains, but he or she will alleviate the recipient's symptoms until a therapist can be contacted. If the woman is having extreme symptoms, she should report them to her midwife or doctor immediately.

1
What is Shiatsu?

Shiatsu is a Japanese acupressure technique the roots of which are in Traditional Chinese Medicine. In the Japanese language, *shi* means "finger" and *atsu* means "pressure", so the word *Shiatsu* means "finger pressure". In Shiatsu, however, the knees, elbows and feet are also used for applying pressure on the body.

In Shiatsu, specific points called tsubos, located along the body's meridians, are manipulated very much as for acupuncture, in order to produce balance in the energy flow. This energy flow is called Qi, pronounced "*chee*", and is alternatively referred to as Chi, Chee or Ki.

The thirteen meridians and the abbreviations I have chosen to use for them in this book are listed in Table 1.1.

Table 1.1
The meridians and their abbreviations

Meridian	Abbreviation
Bladder	BL
Conception Vessel	CV
Gallbladder	GB
Governing Vessel	GV
Heart	HT
Kidney	KID
Large Intestine	LI
Liver	LIV
Lung	LU
Pericardium	PC
Small Intestine	SI
Spleen	SP
Stomach	ST
Triple Warmer (Triple Heater)	TW

The Shiatsu therapist can redress imbalances in movement of Qi that occur in the form of blockage, reversal or deficiency. I describe these three conditions as follows.

Blockage of Qi

This can cause pain as a result of build-up of Qi and inability of body Fluids to flow along the meridians and other channels such as Blood vessels.

Reversal of Qi, or Rebellious Qi

As suggested in its two names, this is movement of Qi against the normal flow. A very good example of reversal of Qi is morning sickness, or pregnancy nausea, whereby Stomach Qi, which usually flows down normally, is reversed – or rebels – and results in vomiting.

Deficiency of Qi

This can cause pain when Qi, Blood or Fluids are insufficient for feeding the body's needs.

These three conditions can be caused by environmental, musculoskeletal, dietary and/or emotional factors. The Shiatsu therapist considers all three conditions when he or she is treating the recipient.

Of the many types of Shiatsu, the four most commonly used are Zen Shiatsu, Namikoshi-style Shiatsu, Barefoot Shiatsu and Jin Shin Do, which I describe as follows.

I Zen Shiatsu

In this type of Shiatsu, the therapist uses "setu-shin" techniques whereby he or she makes a diagnosis by touching the recipient in order to balance and harmonise Yin and Yang. The therapist uses the Chinese meridian system as well as meridians specifically used in Zen Shiatsu.

2 Namikoshi-style Shiatsu

The roots of this type of Shiatsu are in Traditional Chinese Medicine as well as in osteopathy. The therapist adopts a more Western-style approach to diagnosis, and uses only his or her hands and fingers to apply pressure to the recipient's body.

3 Barefoot Shiatsu

As the name suggests, in this type of Shiatsu the therapist uses mainly his or her feet to apply pressure to the recipient's body. Barefoot Shiatsu is a very deep and penetrating technique, and can be dangerous if the therapist has not been properly trained to apply it.

4 Jin Shin Do

In the Japanese language, *jin* means "compassion", *shin* means "spirit", and *do* means "the way". Jin Shin Do can be compared to the reiki technique, whereby the therapist maintains a barely detectable, light, soft pressure on the recipient's body for only a short time. The two techniques benefit both the therapist and the recipient.

In all types of Shiatsu, the therapist supplements pressure application with stretches and rotations. Shiatsu is a holistic therapy because the therapist considers the recipient's diet and lifestyle and incorporates both of them in diagnosis and treatment.

Traditionally, the Shiatsu recipient is fully clothed in loose, natural clothing and undergoes the treatment on a futon on the floor. The therapist's treatment techniques can be either specific to a style of Shiatsu or a combination of styles, as appropriate for the recipient. It is very important that the therapist maintain both flow and integration when applying his or her technique so that calm and harmony can be maintained during the treatment session.

Glossary

Following is a glossary of the special terms that recur throughout the book.

Blood[1]	Blood's four main activities in the body are to circulate continuously, to nourish, to maintain and to moisten. Because it is liquid, it is considered to be a Yin substance.
Fluids[2]	Fluids are liquids other than Blood. Their function in the body is to moisten and nourish the bones, brain, flesh, hair, joints, marrow, membranes, muscles, organs and skin.
Hara	The Hara is the body's physical centre and is located below the navel, in the lower abdomen.
Jiao	The body is divided into three Jiao. The Upper Jiao includes the upper torso, the head and the arms; the Middle Jiao includes the middle torso; and the Lower Jiao includes the pelvic area and the legs.
jitsu	"Jitsu" means the condition of the body, of a point or of the Hara. It indicates excess, fullness, heat and tightness, and is Yang.
kyo	"Kyo" also means the condition of the body, of a point or of the Hara. It indicates deficiency, emptiness, cold and softness, and is Yin.
meridians[3]	Meridians are the body's channels through which Qi flows.
Qi[4]	Qi is the life force, or vital energy, that flows through the meridians.
sedation	Sedation is dispersion or removal of a blockage or stagnation of Qi. It is a more pointed, sharp and quick Shiatsu technique, whereby the therapist uses hard and sustained pressure. The

	therapist usually uses his or her elbows, fists, knees and/or thumbs.
Shen[5]	Shen is the mind, or spirit, and is housed in the heart. It vitalises the body and consciousness and provides the driving force behind the personality. It is reflected in the eyes.
tonification	Tonification is either restoration or putting in of Qi. The therapist usually uses a broader pressure, and a slow and holding technique. He or she usually uses his or her forearms, palms and/or thumbs.
tsubo	Tsubo is the Japanese word for "point". "Tsubo" usually means an acupuncture point on the meridian that can be worked for a specific complaint.
Yin and Yang[6]	To put it simply, Yin and Yang are two polar complements. Using the two words is a convenient way of describing functions of change within the universe, whether the universe is external – environment – or internal – body. Some Yin keywords are chronic, cold, deficient, female, generation of blood, heavy, inactivity, internal, and watery.

Some Yang keywords are activity, acute, dry, excess, expanding, external, hot, light, male, and metabolism.

The traditional graphic representation of Yin and Yang is shown in Figure 1.1. It can be seen that as Yin slowly reduces and becomes Yang, a small amount of it remains in Yang, and vice versa. It is necessary to keep this continuous cycle in harmony in order to have good health.

Figure 1.1 The graphic representation of Yin and Yang.

Information for the therapist and support person

Pregnancy is a normal condition, not an illness. In Traditional Chinese Medicine, the therapist supports the pregnant woman by considering her diet and lifestyle. Many women are very aware of when they conceive and of how their awareness affects the subtle ways in which their body and psyche change. You, the therapist or support person, have to maintain a balance between what you believe to be an appropriate treatment and the pregnant woman's needs.

Although pregnancy is a happy time for most women, in our stressful times the pregnant woman requires much nurturing and support. Shiatsu is a very useful non-intrusive treatment during a woman's pregnancy.

The pregnant woman experiences moments of fear and trepidation about her baby's health. Her fears are natural and are the beginnings of both the mother–child bond and the mother's protective relationship with her child. As a Shiatsu therapist or support person, you are responsible both for understanding that the pregnant woman has to express her natural fears and for acknowledging that expressing her fears is healthy. The woman might voice her concern about conflicting pieces of information she is receiving, such as friends' "old wives' tales" and family members' stories about "bad" experiences of childbirth and pregnancy. She might also be concerned about whether she is eating correctly, about her pre-pregnancy lifestyle and even about whether she is sleeping in the correct position.

Shiatsu is a gentle and nurturing therapy in which the pregnant woman is supported, calmed and relaxed. The Shiatsu therapist supports the woman's antenatal and postnatal care and can be instrumental in procuring a normal birth for her. Although Shiatsu can be used simply to relax the woman, it benefits both her and her baby because it balances Yin and Yang as well as the Blood and Qi.

It is safe to apply Shiatsu techniques to the pregnant woman during all three pregnancy trimesters provided you follow a few simple rules. When you are deciding which treatment to use, always consider the woman and her specific condition. Make sure your intentions are correct and your manner nurturing. As necessary, vary your touch from gentle tonification to sedation, and be mindful that the woman requires both emotional and physical support.

To be an effective therapist or support person during a woman's pregnancy and childbirth, you have to be able to both listen and observe. Your Shiatsu treatment will be appropriate if you

- have a good technique
- are aware of aetiology: the causes of diseases
- are aware of pathology: the symptoms of diseases
- have the intention of being caring and nurturing.

On the following pages, I outline techniques for the woman's antenatal and postnatal care, the complaints that women most commonly suffer both antenatally and postnatally, and the treatment plans for both stages of motherhood. You can enhance the woman's delivery by using Shiatsu and the specific tsubos I include in the text. If you are a support person, you can learn these techniques by systematically reading the applicable sections of the book.

The major aspects of Shiatsu treatment are

1   the treatment-room environment
2   the recipient's position during treatment

3   the Hara
4   concluding the session.

I outline each aspect as follows.

1 The treatment-room environment

Your treatment-room environment should be quiet, clean, warm and private. Listening to gentle music can be soothing, although it isn't necessary to play music. Always ask the recipient what her needs are with reference to music, use of the mat, her position and room temperature. You can use pillows in order to support the woman's shoulders, lower back, tummy, backs of legs, knees and/or calves. It's therefore a good idea to have ready at least three soft pillows and at least three firm, husk-filled pillows. It can also be useful to have a comfy upright chair.

2 The recipient's position during treatment

As the therapist, you have to be flexible when working with the pregnant woman, because she has to find which position is most comfortable for her. As her middle Jiao becomes heavier, it places strain on her internal organs as well as on her musculoskeletal system. Let her find her own comfortable position, and provide cushions and pillows to support her. You might have to help her lower herself to the mat and raise herself after the treatment. She might prefer to be treated sitting in a chair, so you might find it useful and appropriate to have a sturdy chair in your treatment room. Most pregnant women find lying on their side to be the easiest position for receiving Shiatsu.

3 The Hara

The Hara, or Dan Tien, is located in the lower abdomen, below the navel, and is the body's physical centre. Because the Shiatsu recipient is positioned on the floor and the therapist is usually on his or hands and knees, the Hara provides the therapist with a balanced centre of gravity.

In the Hara are incorporated the Yin, or Earth, flowing up the front of the body, and the Yang, or Heaven, flowing down the back of the body into the lower abdomen.

The main concept of Shiatsu is that the treatment flows from the therapist's Hara. Therefore, by focussing all your attention and movement to be from this centre of gravity, you are assured of treating the recipient in a harmonious and supportive way. Because you are using your Hara as your centre of gravity, you can use your body weight and not only your hand and arm muscles to dictate pressure. For you, Shiatsu is therefore less tiring than other body-work techniques and an almost meditative effect is thereby created. When it is used correctly, Shiatsu benefits both therapist and recipient.

If you always work your treatment from the Hara, you will never damage the recipient. Do not allow your head – your mentality and physicality – to overrule your Hara. Your whole treatment is supported when you keep your Hara in total energetic contact with your recipient's Hara. You achieve total contact of both Haras by making sure your body position adjusts itself to that of your recipient. You and your treatment are grounded when you work from the Hara. If your centre of gravity is always from the Hara, you reduce excess pressure on points, and a more appropriate energy release occurs.

According to Endo Ryokyo in his book *Tao Shiatsu*,

Healers must be careful not to use only the weight of the top half of their body when leaning on the patient, because doing so will gradually exhaust their own ki. This is because the weight of the top part of the body and that of the lower part of the body are separate, and when applying pressure the movement of the body must work as a whole. It is best to lean with the upper part of the body while visualising leaning with the weight of the lower part of the body. By doing this, the healer's whole body weight is in contact with the patient, enabling the appropriate application of steady, continuous pressure and ensuring that the healer's ki is not exhausted.[7]

To direct yourself during treatment, use your Hara, not your head, legs or arms: the former method is much less tiring for you and much more beneficial to the recipient. I find it helps to visualise an energy connection or even a cord that connects me to the recipient through our navels. If my navel is in a direct line with my recipient's navel, a strong connection between the two Haras is created. If, for example, you are working at the recipient's head, position yourself kneeling behind her and make a direct line by being consciously aware of where your Hara is in relation to your recipient's Hara. I let the two haras "pull" towards and away from each other. If you are working from the side, you might find it easier to have one of your knees upraised and your other leg supporting, whereby you can again visualise the two Haras as being connected by an invisible cord.

4 Concluding the treatment

When you have completed your treatment, it is appropriate to take your leave by letting the recipient know you are finished. I usually suggest he or she lie there on the futon for a while. When you think it appropriate to do so, ask how the woman is feeling and suggest she can now slowly roll to her side then sit up, ready to leave. Do not rush this part of the session, and in your schedule allow for at least five to ten minutes of recovery time. If I have been playing music during the session, I gently reduce the volume to nil; doing so is a good indicator that the session is over and that the recipient may start to get up.

It is of no use having a good technique or knowing about points, stretches and pressure if there is no intention of care and support. Likewise, if you know about aetiology and pathology but are lacking in care, you do not help the recipient to relax and help you in your treatment. If you have the intention of being caring and supportive; have a good technique; know about points, stretches and pressure; and know about aetiology and pathology, you will achieve optimal results for the recipient. Shiatsu is a therapy in which the emotional, physical and mental are blended with knowledge, touch, intention, and dietary and lifestyle recommendations. Throughout the book, I indicate specific tsubos or points as a formula for clearing the pathology.

Caution

Although the following seven points can be used during the third trimester of pregnancy both in preparation for and during birth, they are too strong to use during the first two trimesters.

1	Bladder 60	(BL60)
2	Bladder 63	(BL63)
3	Gallbladder 21	(GB21)
4	Lower Intestine 4	(LI4)
5	Spleen 6	(SP6)
6	Spleen 9	(SP9)
7	Stomach 36	(ST36)

These seven contraindicated points are very strong, because they are used in order to descend (draw down) Qi, so it is understandable that their use is banned during early pregnancy. Because they are descending points, if they are used inappropriately they can cause miscarriage, especially if the woman's Qi is deficient.

Throughout the book, I indicate when these points can be used for specific conditions. When this is the case, I also suggest techniques whereby they can be used safely. Because it is very strong and can cause a strong descending effect, Barefoot Shiatsu is not usually indicated for use during pregnancy.

Further on in the book, I suggest some dietary adjustments and exercises for the recipient to learn and undertake at home, as an adjunct to the Shiatsu techniques.

2
Pregnancy physiology: Traditional Chinese Medicine

During a woman's pregnancy, maintaining Qi and Blood flow as well as balancing Yin and Yang are the main areas of concern. Balancing Yin and Yang is important because of the balancing as a whole that it represents. There cannot be either Yin without Yang or Yang without Yin.

For the foetus to form, this balance of the parents' duality – the male Yang and the female Yin – is required because of the wholeness of duality. The foetus's formation can be upset by either deficiency or excess of Yin or Yang. Yin symbolises the denser forms of material, Yang the rarefied forms of it, so the two combine to form a healthy person. According to Giovanni Maciocia in his book *The Foundations of Chinese Medicine*,

> Yin is quiet, Yang is active. Yang gives life, Yin makes it grow. Yang is transformed into Qi, Yin is transformed into material life.[8]

Tai Kyo

The health of the embryo and foetus is determined by the balance between Heaven and Earth, Water and Fire, and Yin and Yang. In Traditional Chinese Medicine, education of the embryo and foetus is called Tai Kyo. According to the authors Waturo Ohashi and Mary M. Hoover in their book *Natural Childbirth, the Eastern Way*,

> It is traditionally thought in the Orient that that one third of a person's ultimate social, physical and mental functioning is determined by his or her experiences in the womb. So tai kyo is very important.[9]

The pregnant woman's experiences that would benefit the foetus are receiving Shiatsu, listening to soothing rather than jarring music, being relaxed and happy rather than angry, and eating healthy food. Naturally, it is believed that the foetus would be unbeneficially affected by the woman's ingesting drugs or alcohol, listening to jarring music, being consistently upset or experiencing extreme emotional states.

Pre-Heaven and Post-Heaven Essence

With reference to Blood, Qi is Yang, and Blood is a denser form of Qi and is therefore Yin. Qi has the specifically Yang qualities of warming, protecting, transforming and raising; blood has the specifically Yin qualities of nourishing and moistening. According to Giovanni Maciocia,

> A human being results from the Qi of Heaven and Earth . . . The union of the Qi of Heaven and Earth is called a human being.[10]

Conception occurs when a man's and woman's sexual energies are blended to form "Pre Heaven Essence". Although during pregnancy this essence nourishes the foetus, the essence is dependent on nourishment of the woman's kidneys. According to Maciocia,

The "Pre Heaven Essence" is the only kind of essence present in the foetus, as it does not have independent physiological activity.[11]

We inherit our Pre-Heaven Essence from our parents at conception: it is our constitution and what we will be in life after our birth.

Our "Post-Heaven Essence", which originates in food, exists after we are born, when we suckle and breathe and therefore access the Qi of Spleen, Stomach and Lung.

Whereas we derive our Essence from our parents, our Qi is formed after we are born. Essence controls the child's growth and development both antenatally and postnatally. If the child is to be healthy, functioning and well developed both mentally and physically, it is important he or she have healthy inherited Essence. Essence gives us our constitutional strength to deal with pathogenic resistance and draws its strength from the Kidney Essence to create a functional human being.

Qi and Blood

Although Qi is diverse, it is represented by the basic functions of transporting, holding, raising, protecting and warming.

Although Blood is a form of Qi and is denser and more material, it is Qi. Qi is Blood; Blood is Qi. Qi both enables Blood to flow in the blood vessels, by way of the abovementioned functions of Qi, and transforms into Blood. When we have a good diet, the Spleen and Stomach are enabled to transform and transport, along with Lung Qi, thereby pushing Food Qi to the Heart. Also, the Kidney Essence produces Marrow. Qi's effect on Blood and Blood's effect on Qi are therefore revealed. A strong relationship exists between Qi and Blood: Qi is Yang to Blood, whereas Blood is Yin to Qi.

Qi generates Blood through Food Qi and Lung Qi, moves Blood and holds Blood in the Blood's vessels. Blood nourishes Qi and is therefore known as the Mother of Qi.

We can now recognise the importance of Blood, Qi, and Yin and Yang balance during a woman's pregnancy.

In Traditional Chinese Medicine, the uterus, or womb, is ruled by the ancestral Qi and is known as one of the "extraordinary", or "curious", organs. Traditionally, the uterus and the Eight Extras – the influential points at which Qi and Essence of the eight types of tissue and substance converge – are dependent on metabolism of ancestral Qi by the three Jiao, or the Triple Warmer (also known as the Triple Heater).

- Ren Mai (Figure 2.1) is known as The Conception Vessel (CV), or The Sea of Yin Meridians. It not only regulates the energy flow in all the Yin meridians; it is especially involved in the Qi of the uterus.
- Du Mai (Figure 2.2) is known as The Governing Vessel (GV), or The Sea of Blood. It is related to the pelvic cavity, and regulates Qi and Blood in all the twelve meridians.
- Dai Mai balances the upper and lower body.
- Yinqiao Mai supports removal of stagnation of Qi and Blood in the lower abdomen, and functions at the level of the genitals.

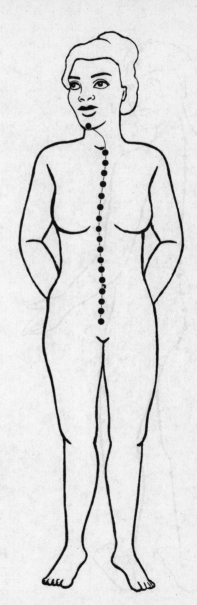

Figure 2.1
Ren Mai: The Conception Vessel (CV),
or The Sea of Yin Meridians.

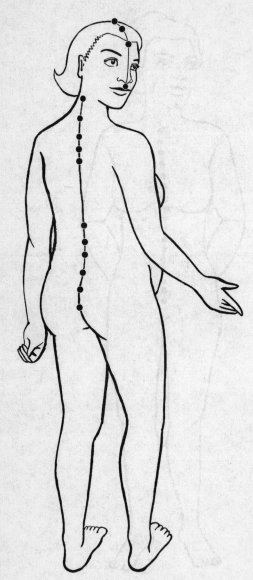

Figure 2.2
Du Mai: The Governing Vessel (GV),
or The Sea of Blood.

In the pelvic cavity, including the uterus, the Blood–Qi balance is negotiated by the thoracic cavity, and both the pelvic cavity and the thoracic cavity are united by Shao Yin, or Heart and Kidney. On the other hand, the Du Mai supplies the Yang to the Yin of both Ren Mai and Du Mai.

With reference to pregnancy, the five most important of the twelve main meridians are as described in Table 2.1.

Table 2.1 The five most important meridians during pregnancy

Meridian	*Abbreviation*	*Description*
Gallbladder	GB	Gallbladder is important because it is associated with the Liver and the Triple Warmer (TW) and because it has a close affinity with the pelvic area.
Heart	HT	Heart is important because the emotions can affect the Heart and can therefore affect the amount of Blood that is available for circulation.
Kidney	KID	Kidney supplies nutritive Qi to the uterus.
Liver	LIV	Liver governs the smooth flow of Qi along with Ren Mai. Du Mai and Liver store the Blood, and Spleen and Liver hold the Blood in its vessels. Liver 9 (LIV9) increases the circulation of Qi to the pelvic cavity.
Spleen	SP	Spleen holds the Blood in the blood vessels. Spleen feeds Blood through the area of the ovaries, and Spleen 10 (SP10: The Sea of Blood) circulates the Blood at this level.

The Connecting and Luo points used in Shiatsu are illustrated in Figure 2.3. Luo points are connecting points between Yin and Yang.

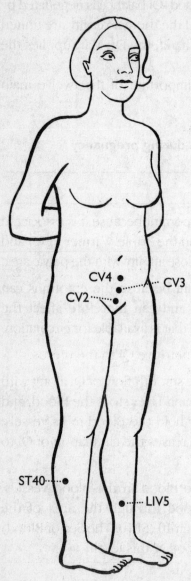

Figure 2.3 The Connecting and Luo points.

The main connections for Kidney are through CV3 (Conception Vessel 3), CV4 and Du Mai; for Liver through CV2, CV3 and CV4; and for Spleen through CV3 and CV4. If there is an imbalance in any of these areas, such as in Kidney Qi, contraction and pain are caused in the genitals. Liver is widely associated with most pain, and Spleen causes a pulling pain in the genitals.

LIV5 (Liver 5), the Luo point of Liver, commands the whole of the genitals, whereas Stomach Luo ST40 aids Spleen in commanding the Blood and is useful for correcting haemorrhage and menstrual irregularity.

3
Pregnancy physiology: the Western way

When a baby girl is born, her ovaries can contain up to 200,000 primary ovarian follicles, which lie in the cortex of the ovary. During the little girl's early years, the activity associated with these follicles is minimal.

When the little girl reaches seven or eight years of age, activity gradually occurs because of a first release of a pituitary hormone called Follicle Stimulating Hormone, or FSH. When this first release of FSH occurs, the primary follicles start to produce small amounts of oestrogen, which gradually increase as the girl ages.

The menstrual cycle
When the girl is somewhere between eleven and sixteen years of age, enough follicles will have been stimulated to maturation. The first ovarian follicle will have ripened to become what is thereafter known as a graafian follicle, and that

follicle will have ruptured to release its ovum, or egg; in other words, the girl's first ovulation will have occurred.

Once the menstrual cycle has been established, several hundred follicles can ripen each month, and each follicle produces an amount of oestrogen. At some stage, one follicle is more mature than the others and produces a larger amount of oestrogen, whereby the other follicles are caused to cease production, atrophy and disappear into the substance of the ovary. This is the stage at which the one follicle that has continued to grow and produce hormones is called a graafian follicle. The process I have described is illustrated in Figure 3.1.

The mature graafian follicle comprises a layer of granulosa cells that surround a space filled with follicular fluid. The ovum is located at one side of this space. When the follicle has matured, it ruptures and thereby expels the ovum into the peritoneal cavity, where it is picked up by the fimbriae of the fallopian tubes.

When the ovum has been released, the cells of the ruptured follicle join together as a ring. Under the influence of luteinising hormone, or LH, as a result of the high levels of oestrogen, the follicle ring forms the corpus luteum. The corpus luteum produces large amounts of progesterone and continues to produce oestrogen. It has a lifespan of between ten and twelve days and is maintained by the hormone human chorionic gonadotrophin, or HCG.

Pregnancy

If the ovum is embedded with a sperm, the lining of the uterus is prepared to support the ovum's growth into a foetus. The changes in the uterine lining respond to production and withdrawal of oestrogen and progesterone.

When menstruation has occurred, the proliferate phase begins. This phase is a time of repair and rebuilding, whereby tiny blood vessels swell with blood, and continues until ovulation occurs. Once ovulation occurs and progesterone levels rise, the glands of the endometrium become activated and start to secrete mucus, glycogen and other substances. This process occurs specifically to aid the

Figure 3.1
The menstrual cycle: maturation of the follicle and ovum, release of the
ovum, and degeneration of the follicle should pregnancy not have resulted
after ovulation.

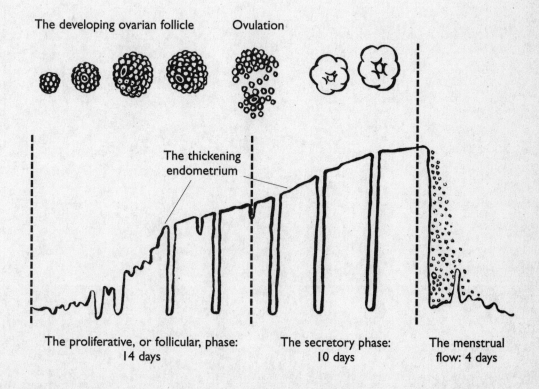

The developing ovarian follicle   Ovulation

The thickening
endometrium

The proliferative, or follicular, phase:
14 days

The secretory phase:
10 days

The menstrual
flow: 4 days

fertilised ovum's embedding and nourishment and is called the secretory phase. If all is well and progesterone maintains the oestrogen levels, the fertilised ovum is embedded in the endometrium and pregnancy commences with the first sign of amenorrhea, or absence of menstruation.

4
Taking the pregnant woman's history

As a Shiatsu therapist, you have to take a full, pre-pregnancy history of your recipient's menstrual cycle before she was pregnant in order to identify any pregnancy-related problems that might occur.

A normal menstrual cycle lasts between twenty-six and thirty-two days; the average time is twenty-eight days. The blood flow lasts for up to between four and six days and gradually decreases during the last day or two. Clotting, pain, bloating and distension should be either minimal or absent. A healthy blood flow is neither brown nor muddy. Most women experience a dragging sensation and/or cramping before their menses, or periods, begin. Headaches and extreme cravings for sweets should be absent, and the woman should not feel depleted because her menses are beginning or have begun.

Ideally, the Shiatsu recipient will have prepared for her pregnancy by adjusting her lifestyle and diet. However, the reality is that many recipients find they are pregnant and have one or more conditions that if not treated might affect the pregnancy, the woman and the foetus.

...n you are taking the woman's history, examine her pre-pregnancy ...rual cycle by looking for the three conditions and their symptoms as listed in Table 4.1.

Table 4.1
The three conditions and their symptoms

Condition	Symptoms
Liver Qi Stagnation	Dark blood, blood clots, pain and pre-menstrual tension (PMT). Liver Qi stagnation might cause morning sickness, miscarriage or eclampsia (a type of epileptic convulsion caused by anatomical lesion, or damage) during the pregnancy.
Blood Deficiency	Vertigo (dizziness), emaciation (thinness and feebleness), blurred vision, numbness of the extremities (hands and feet), dry skin and hair, and/or face paleness. Blood Deficiency might cause miscarriage, eclampsia or haemorrhaging during the pregnancy.
Rising Liver Qi	Headaches and excessive bleeding. If Stagnant Fire is present, the woman has heat in her breast area, is excessively thirsty, might have leukorrhea (an unusual vaginal discharge) and might even have a red complexion. Rising Liver Qi might cause miscarriage, depression, insomnia or spotting (loss of small amounts of blood through the vagina) during the pregnancy.

Miscarriage

All three conditions described in the table might indicate that miscarriage is possible, so you have to consider the issues associated with miscarriage when you are treating the woman. Many first pregnancies end in miscarriage because the foetus is unviable, a fact that could be viewed as being nature's way of dealing with a non-viable pregnancy. Sometimes nothing can be done to save the pregnancy, in which case the woman might require counselling, have her grief accepted and be generally reassured.

Habitual miscarriage can result when Spleen Qi is insufficient for holding the foetus within the uterus, when there is Heat in the Blood or when there is Blood Deficiency. All three conditions respond favourably to Shiatsu, whereby the foetus reaches full term. Other problems can occur during pregnancy as a result of the three conditions, so if possible, use your diagnosis and treatment to pre-empt any future problems.

Diet

It is important that the woman have a good diet during her pregnancy. Her energy has to be optimised early in the pregnancy so that she enjoys her new state.

When you are suggesting to the woman that she make therapeutic changes to her diet, consider her current eating habits and incorporate in your suggestions any foods she likes to eat. If her diet does not include macrobiotic or even Chinese foods, carefully consider her own food choices when you are suggesting dietary therapy.

I find that soups are a food that most people enjoy and are able to incorporate easily in their diet. If the woman is eating cold or raw foods, explain how it is necessary for the pregnant woman to nurture the foetus by instead eating warm and well-digested foods. Describe how digestion of cold or raw foods depletes Qi, or energy, and thereby requires the Qi and Blood to be strengthened.

Lifestyle

The woman's lifestyle is another important factor for you to consider, because any physical or emotional stress should be reduced. If the woman is highly stressed, offer options that will help her reduce the stress. Suggest she practise Hara breathing, yoga and Tai Chi, and for more suggestions, refer to "Chapter 10: Exercise therapy" in this book.

Devise for the woman a simple exercise plan through which Qi is strengthened, back pain is alleviated, the hips are strengthened and loosened, and the perineum is stretched. Introduce only one exercise during each treatment session in order to build up a good exercise regimen that the woman will find easy to learn and practise.

Explain to the woman the effects on both herself and the foetus of smoking, alcohol and drugs and how it is necessary for her to conserve her Qi and Blood. However, let her make her own decisions about these matters: support and nurture her but do not moralise about any "bad habits" she might have.

Pulse and tongue

Examining the woman's tongue gives you a good indication of the health of both the woman and the foetus. Examining the pulse effectively indicates the condition of Qi and the Blood, and examining the tongue might aid you in diagnosing presence of Heat and/or Damp as well as the state of both Qi and the Blood.

Other key indicators

Three other indicators of the woman's health are the quality of her bowel movements, the quality of her urine and her sleep patterns.

Expectations

Ask the woman what her expectations are with reference to Shiatsu treatment. Personally, I prefer to treat the presenting problems in order to give the woman relief in those areas.

The support person's role in taking the woman's history

If you are the woman's support person, you will have to ask her some simple questions in order to ensure you are aware of any needs and painful bodily areas with reference to her treatment position and your Shiatsu pressure.

It is also useful if you know about any symptoms so you can decide which points – tsubos – to use during the session. Always be observant of the woman's physical condition: look for face paleness, lethargy, a voice that is unusually soft, any breathing problems, imbalance in weightbearing during walking and the woman's general state of health.

Face paleness can be caused by Blood Deficiency or Qi Deficiency. Lethargy can be caused by Spleen Qi disharmony or Qi Deficiency in general. An unusually soft voice and breathing problems can indicate Lung Qi disharmony. Imbalance in weightbearing whereby one bodily part is used more, as in the case of leaning more on one leg, can indicate presence of pain in the side opposite to the favoured bodily part. Although you might not be able to make a total diagnosis, having a general idea about which meridian is in disharmony will aid you with reference to what your intention will be during the session.

Pregnancy signs and symptoms

The pulse

Differences in the woman's pulse rate can aid you in detecting whether she is pregnant: you will feel her pulse to be a "rolling", or "slippery", Spleen pulse. The pulse rate is used for determining whether Yin Blood is deficient, excessive, hot or cold. The correct position for taking your recipient's pulse is illustrated in Figure 4.1, and the three pulses on each wrist are illustrated in Figure 4.2.

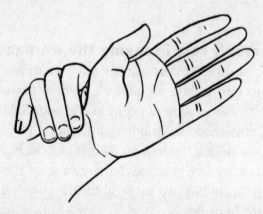

Figure 4.1 The correct position for taking your recipient's pulse.

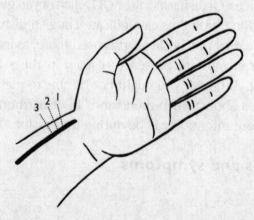

Figure 4.2 The three pulses on each wrist,
as distinguished in Traditional Chinese Medicine.

Because the foetus is formed from Jing and is nourished by blood, pregnancy can be detected on the Shao Yin pulse at the Cun position of the left hand: the beat comes and goes and is almost slippery. The pulse at the Chi and Guan positions can seem to be smooth and slippery.

The Cun position belongs to the Heart meridian (HT), which controls the blood vessels, and the Chi position belongs to the Kidney meridian (KID), which stores Jing. For a viable foetus to be formed, Jing and Blood have to be in harmony.

During the third and fourth months of pregnancy, the pulse at the Chi position is slippery and rapid, and if pressure is applied it can become soft and scattered. During approximately the fifth month, although the pulse remains slippery and rapid, if pressure is applied it is no longer soft and scattered.

Interestingly, feeling the woman's pulse can determine whether the foetus is male or female. However, I have found this method to be only about 70 per cent accurate. If the foetus is male, the Chi pulse of the woman's left hand seems to be more slippery and rapid than that of her right, and her abdomen is swollen as in the base of a wok. If the foetus is female, the Chi pulse of the woman's right hand seems to be more slippery and rapid than that of her left, and her abdomen is the shape of a "bamboo wheelbarrow".[12]

These two types of pulse are easily detected during the fifth and sixth months of pregnancy, at which time the abdominal shape can be observed easily. I do not make this method of determining the baby's sex available to my Shiatsu recipients unless they ask whether a sex-determining method exists. If you detect the abovementioned pulse characteristics and decide to reveal the baby's likely sex to your recipient, I suggest you also point out the 30 per cent error factor in the method's accuracy.

Other pregnancy indicators

Other indicators that a woman is pregnant are cessation of her menses, increase in her vaginal secretions, increase in her appetite, vertigo (dizziness), fatigue, nausea, enlargement and sensitisation of her breasts, and sometimes presence of a crampy backache around her hips. Other indicators might be frequency of urination, slight constipation and slightly elevated temperature.

Although cessation of menses is a good indicator that a woman is pregnant, some pregnant women might have a slight "show" (blood from the vagina) every month. In Western medicine, this "show" is not considered to be a problem if no other symptoms, such as pelvic pain, are present. In Traditional Chinese Medicine, however, the possibility that Spleen Qi is not holding, perhaps because of prevalence of a Damp condition before the woman became pregnant, might have to be considered.

Pregnancy length and the three trimesters

Typically, the length of a pregnancy is between thirty-eight and forty-two weeks, or between 280 and 288 days, and the estimated date of delivery (EDD) is calculated from the last normal menstrual period (LNMP). The EDD is not calculated from the date of conception, because that date cannot be determined with any certainty.

Pregnancy is divided into three trimesters, or three-month segments, and the length of each trimester is approximately thirteen weeks: 3 trimesters multiplied by 13 weeks equals a 39- to 40-week pregnancy.

The first trimester: weeks 1 to 13

At this stage the growing baby is called the embryo, and it is the most delicate stage because the quality of the rest of the pregnancy is established during it. You should advise the newly pregnant woman to totally abstain from alcohol, drugs and tobacco if she has not done so already.

My newly pregnant Shiatsu recipients sometimes tell me their friends have suggested drinking raspberry-leaf tea because it is "good for pregnancy". I tell these women to avoid drinking the tea during the first trimester because doing so aids uterine contractions; they should therefore wait until the third trimester.

Morning sickness

During the first trimester, demand is placed on Liver, Kidney and Spleen Qi. Many women experience morning sickness, which is a misnomer because the feelings of sickness can occur in the evening or throughout the day, not only in the morning.

Most women experience morning sickness as nausea, and some women experience it as vomiting and/or dizziness. It is considered to result from one of the following three problems.

1   Rising of Liver Qi, the symptoms of which can be acidic vomiting, regurgitating, belching, having a bitter taste in the mouth and having a congested chest
2   Rebelling upwards of Yang Qi, the symptoms of which are being excessively thirsty, vomiting, feeling dizzy, suffering tinnitus (ringing in the ears), being insomniac, experiencing heart palpitations and having a congested chest
3   Obstruction of the stomach by Phlegm-Damp, the symptoms of which are acidic regurgitating, vomiting a watery substance, feeling dizzy, experiencing heart palpitations, having a congested chest and finding food to be tasteless

The second trimester: weeks 14 to 26

From this stage onwards the baby is called the foetus, and the woman's abdomen becomes noticeably enlarged. For most women, morning sickness subsides, usually because the bodily and Qi changes have balanced out and the woman seems to be more content and relaxed.

The woman feels the foetus quickening, or fluttering, as his or her movements become more distinct.

It is now appropriate to review the woman's lifestyle and diet and to suggest she make changes in advance of the third trimester.

The third trimester: weeks 27 to 39–40

The third and final trimester is a time of growth for the foetus. Late in the trimester, he or she moves into the birth position, which is usually head down in order to enter the birth canal (vagina).

The woman might experience lower-back pain, have painful hips, be constipated, have some urinary incontinence and notice small uterine contractions known as Braxton Hicks contractions.

That the baby's birth is imminent is indicated by presence of paroxysmal (wave-like) abdominal contractions, which are usually experienced as a downward pressure in the lower abdomen. As the uterus contracts more and more, the woman experiences ever stronger downward pressure in the lumbar and abdominal regions, and shorter intervals between contractions.

5
Shiatsu treatment
for the pregnant woman

I address this chapter to the trained Shiatsu therapist. However, if you are the recipient's (untrained) support person, you will also find it useful, because I list easily identifiable therapy methods under the heading "A suggested treatment for the support person to apply". When I refer to the recipient, I use the feminine pronouns "she" and "her" in view of the fact that the book is about Shiatsu for the pregnant woman.

If you are the support person, when you read the first section of the chapter, about treatments for the first, second and third trimesters, you should know that you might be unable to meet all the treatment criteria I discuss.

After this first section, I present a section headed "Some important considerations with reference to applying any Shiatsu treatment".

At the end of the important considerations, I illustrate both three correct and three incorrect positions for the therapist and support person to be aware of.

then move on to describe and illustrate the two basic Shiatsu techniques of palming and thumbing.

Finally, I present and illustrate a simple but effective treatment under the heading "A basic Shiatsu session for the support person to conduct". This treatment is safe for the pregnant woman to undergo during any and all of the three trimesters. It is not pregnancy specific; indeed, once you have perfected it, you will find it benefits both adult recipients and child recipients who are more than ten years of age.

The first trimester

Your recipient's treatment position

At this stage of pregnancy, most women find that the position they adopt during treatment is not important. Many can tolerate lying on both their tummy and their back. Some have bouts of extreme morning sickness whereby their abdominal area is sensitive to both touch and pressure.

Always ask the recipient whether she would prefer to lie on her side. If she does, use pillows to support her legs and if necessary her back. I find that rice-husk pillows are useful because they provide support without being too soft, can be shaped to the recipient's body and are light and therefore easily moved during the treatment. The first trimester is the most sensitive time of pregnancy because the embryo is slowly forming and is susceptible to both internal and external variants.

Contraindicated substances

Many medications as well as substances such as tobacco, alcohol and recreational drugs are contraindicated at this stage. For some women it can be a time of emotional turmoil, and for others there is the fear they did the wrong things up to the time they discovered they were pregnant. Now is the time to reassure the Shiatsu recipient. Although she might have read a lot of information about the ill-effects of some substances, she requires support from you during her pregnancy. You should not withdraw your support if the pregnant woman has decided to continue using an unsuitable substance. According to Endo Ryokyo in *Tao Shiatsu*,

> The work of the Shiatsu Therapist is not to correct or change patients but to wholly accept their life through reading their responses to pressure and to allow them the freedom of self expression. Becoming passive toward patients means accepting their individual existence wholly and not measuring it by other standards.[13]

You should neither scold nor impose your own morality on the woman if she has used or is continuing to use a substance that is contraindicated during pregnancy. Reassure her that she can rectify most of her unhealthy habits and that you will support her in making her own decisions. Inform her that either moderating or reducing these habits can be beneficial for her.

As Shiatsu therapists it is not our place to condemn our pregnant recipients: we have to support them and treat them in a way whereby we promote the health of both them and their baby. Personally, I believe that in this context our role is to support the woman and offer suggestions; it is her right to either incorporate or not incorporate our ideas in her lifestyle.

The major points contraindicated during the first trimester
During the first trimester, you should not use the contraindicated points BL60, BL63, GB21, LI4, SP6, SP9 and ST36, which are illustrated in Figure 5.1: they are strong descending, or drawing-down, points.

Figure 5.1
The major points contraindicated during the first trimester.

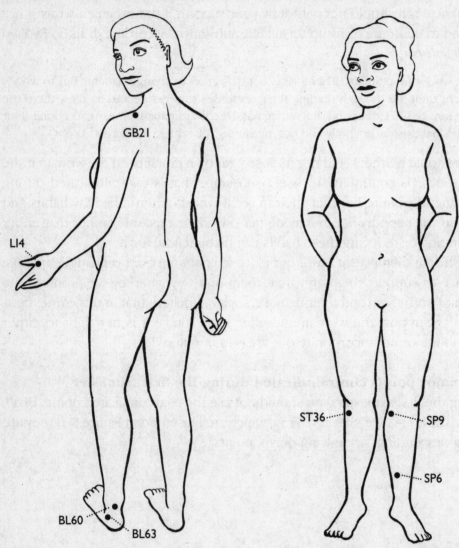

If your recipient is complaining she has neck and shoulder ache, you can work the Gallbladder meridian by using stretching and tonification techniques.

Some women complain they have a dragging or pulling sensation or a short, slightly sharp pain in their pelvic area. These sensations are normal because at this time the uterus and pelvis are adjusting to the foetus and the changing levels of hormones. Naturally, if the woman is having a discharge of either blood or fluid, you should advise her to immediately consult her midwife or doctor.

Lower-back ache

For the first trimester, I find that pregnant women obtain relief from lower-back ache when I sedate the sacral (lower-back bone) area. You should sedate the recipient's Bladder meridian down her back and legs, and emphasise the points Chengfu BL36 and Chengshan BL57. When you are stretching your recipient in this way, both stretch each shoulder away from the hip and do the shoulders-crossover stretch. Also stretch the points BL12 to BL32 inclusive.

Know whether the woman has any deficiency: it probably results from a previous delivery.

Moxabustion

Please refer to "Appendix 1: Moxabustion" on pages 112–14 of *Chinese Medicine for Women*. Moxabustion, or moxa, is a common treatment method whereby localised heat is applied to points of specific parts of the body. It is highly recommended for cases of deficiency, and when applied to Mingmen and Yongquan KID1 it is very beneficial for strengthening the Kidney meridian.

The Gallbladder (GB) meridian

During the first trimester, the point GB30 can be tender and jitsu; if so, use elbow pressure and palming to help stretch it. If the woman has aching hip joints, you greatly relieve her pain if you stretch and even sedate GB30.

At this stage, you should be wary about treating the point GB31: it is usually an Ah Shi (painful) point and can be sensitive to strong pressure. If this is the case, you can use sweeping and palming down the Gallbladder meridian in order to remove any stagnation.

Treating the woman's hips helps relieve tension in her shoulders and neck. Tonify the point GB41 by doing stretching and pulling.

The points GB14 and GB19 and the temporal sides of the pregnant woman's head are three other Gallbladder areas you can work in order to help relieve neck and shoulder tension. It can be useful to work GB25 in order to alleviate vomiting associated with morning sickness.

The Liver (LIV) meridian

During the first trimester, you should tonify, not sedate, Liver points. The Liver meridian is active during the second half of the menstrual cycle. It has been found to promote the level of progesterone,[14] and progesterone creates a viable environment for the fertilised egg to adhere to the endometrium. You should tonify Liver in order to promote holding of Blood, because sedating it might move Blood too strongly and thereby cause miscarriage.

At this stage, Liver is very sensitive to the touch, so you should palm and stretch gently.

The Spleen (SP) meridian

During the first trimester, Spleen is also very sensitive to the touch, so it is also appropriate to gently palm and stretch for this reason. You give the pregnant woman a good Spleen stretch by palming and stretching *up* the Spleen meridian, by gently pushing out her ankles, legs and hips.

The Heart (HT) meridian

You should incorporate the Heart meridian in your first-trimester treatment, because at this stage most pregnant women have bouts of vagueness and lack concentration. During pregnancy, the Heart has to work harder in order to create blood for feeding both the baby and the woman. As more blood is being channelled to the developing baby, the woman suffers slight Blood Deficiency, whereby she becomes vague and unable to concentrate.

The Hara

During the first trimester, your work on the Hara has to be gentle and nurturing. You should not work it very deeply, because if you do, the woman might feel invaded and distressed. Personally, I prefer to undertake Jin Shin Do by holding my left palm over the point CV4 and using my right hand to hold CV6. I then move my right hand to CV16 in order to harmonise the Conception Vessel (CV).

Your recipient's response

Always be aware of your recipient's response to your touch, and adjust your treatment to suit her needs. During the treatment, you might find it useful to ask your recipient to comment on whether your pressure is too hard – or even too soft.

The second trimester

Your recipient's treatment position

At this stage, you might find your recipient prefers to be treated lying on her side. If this is the case, use a pillow to support her upper leg, place a "peanut" pillow or rolled-up towel under her lower hip, and if necessary place a pillow under her breasts.

When your recipient is lying on her back, it might also be necessary to place a pillow under her knees in order to remove pressure from the lower back. At the time of writing, many Western doctors were suggesting that for pregnant women, lying on the back causes obstruction on the aorta and femoral arteries. Personally, I believe that if you limit the woman's lying-down time to ten or fifteen minutes you will not cause harm. If the woman is uncomfortable about lying on her back at all, do not force the issue.

Finish your second-trimester treatment by having your recipient either sit in a chair or continue to lie on her side.

The pulse rate

During the second trimester, you might feel the woman's pulse to be intermittent. The reasons it is intermittent are that Yuan Qi is failing and that Channel Qi is not communicating with Mai Qi. This blockage can also lead to Damp. In your treatment, it is appropriate you support Spleen and Kidney through tonification. Also, Triple Warmer tonification is appropriate for facilitating an even flow of Fluids through the three Jiao.

The Bladder (BL) meridian

Your recipient might feel her developing baby as heaviness on her back and internal organs. In this case, the Bladder meridian is usually stiff and aching, and you might find several stagnant points along it. The restriction of Qi flow is caused by the fact that the foetus is growing in size in the woman's pelvic area.

During Shiatsu treatment, many pregnant women respond quickly to Qi movement, especially that down the Kidney meridian and/or the Bladder meridian. Take this fact into consideration, because you have to work neither too long nor too strongly on either meridian in order to achieve movement and a good Qi flow.

achieve the turn. You can teach the woman to treat herself in this way if it is not convenient for her to be treated by you every day.

Once the baby has turned, the moxa ceases. Although most women are aware their baby is turning, your recipient might wish to have the process verified by her midwife or doctor. The baby can breech several times, in which case you or your recipient can use moxa in order to help the baby turn to the correct position. This use of the moxa treatment has excellent results, and I promote it whenever I believe it is necessary.

Use of contraindicated points

During the two weeks before the estimated date of delivery, if the woman requests it I use the major contraindicated points BL60, BL63, GB21, LI4, SP6, SP9 and ST36 in order to prepare her for an easy labour and birth.

You should use these points carefully and consider any health problems the woman has. *If you have any doubts at all about using the points, do not use them.*

During the final two weeks of the woman's pregnancy, you can use gentle pressure to treat these points once a week. The woman cannot tolerate strong pressure because the points can be very sensitive and painful.

Lower-back ache

During the third trimester, most women feel a general ache in their lower back, in which case it helps to apply either moxa or a heat pack to the area. You should not advise your recipient to use cold packs on the area, because they contribute to invasion of cold whereby problems can be created for the woman both during labour and after the birth. During the third trimester, the three most common problems are presence of cold-type pain, constriction of Blood flow and constriction of Qi flow.

Some important considerations
with reference to applying any Shiatsu treatment

- Shiatsu treatment is relaxing and calming, and your recipient's body temperature could drop during your session. In your treatment room, maintain a comfortable temperature for your recipient and have a blanket nearby in case she requests it.
- At the start of your session, take five minutes to calm and still your mind by breathing deeply into your Hara. Become aware of your mind, and breathe directly into your Hara. When you are Hara breathing, while you are calming yourself you might find it helpful to put your hands on either side of your navel.
- During your session, maintain awareness of your breathing, and remain relaxed and calm.
- Consider your recipient's specific needs and that you intend to cause her no harm. When you consider her in this way, your touch will be relevant and appropriate.
- Always maintain contact with your recipient, mentally and/or physically. Devote yourself to her. When you are, for example, using one of your hands to work one of your recipient's legs, you should hold your other hand on her body so you maintain contact. During your treatment, your non-moving hand is known as the mother hand.
- Watch your recipient for any reaction she might have to the pressure you are applying. Her reactions can include holding her breath, tightening her muscles and screwing up her face or eyes. When your recipient's reaction indicates she is feeling pain, you should adjust your pressure. Talk to your recipient, and check whether you are applying your pressure either too firmly or too deeply.
- Move your recipient's limbs and head slowly, and if necessary let her move into a comfortable position. Do not force any part of her body.

- Take your time. If after one hour you have not followed all the directions on this checklist, do not be concerned, because the power of touch is the most important aspect of any Shiatsu therapy.
- Rest on your toes in order to take the weight off your knees, and alternate from your left knee to your right knee. Use your legs, not your arms, to push off. Practise these techniques on a pillow before you start working on a Shiatsu recipient.

Correct and incorrect positions

The photo pairs in figures 5.2, 5.3 and 5.4 illustrate the positions you should adopt and avoid when you are conducting a Shiatsu treatment.

In Figure 5.2b, the therapist's body is too close to her hands, whereby her back becomes hunched and her shoulders lifted. She would probably suffer lower-back ache were she to use this position and would not be able to easily lean into her recipient. Her feet are flat and she is not supporting her legs on her toes, so she would probably have pain in her legs and knees.

Figure 5.2a
*The first **correct** position for the therapist or support person to adopt.*

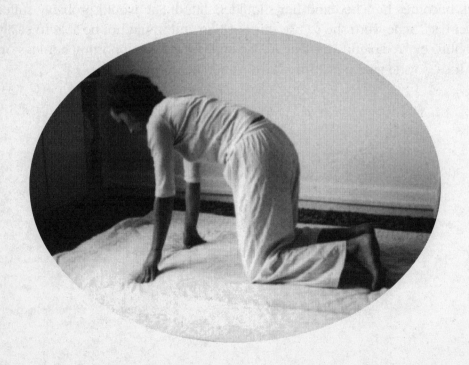

Figure 5.2b
The first incorrect position.

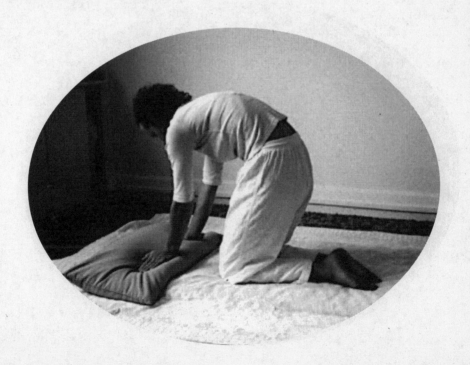

In Figure 5.3b, the therapist is leaning too far forward over her recipient. Also, her feet are flat, and she is not supporting her legs on her toes. Her recipient would find the therapist's pressure to be uncomfortable. The therapist would tire quickly and have sore arms after only a short time.

Figure 5.3a
*The second **correct** position.*

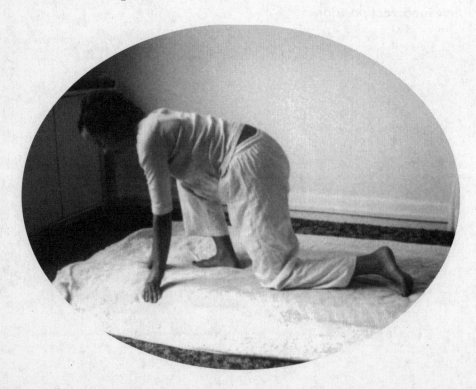

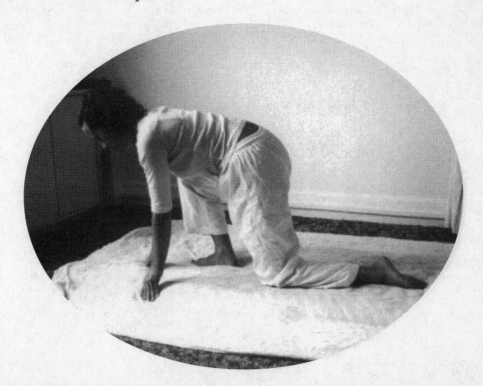

Figure 5.3b
*The second **incorrect** position.*

In Figure 5.4b, the therapist is again too close to her recipient. The position of her hara, or centre of gravity, is incorrect for enabling her to easily lean into her recipient. Were she to use this position, her lower back would take a lot of strain and she would thereby have either pain or aching.

Figure 5.4a
The third **correct** *position.*

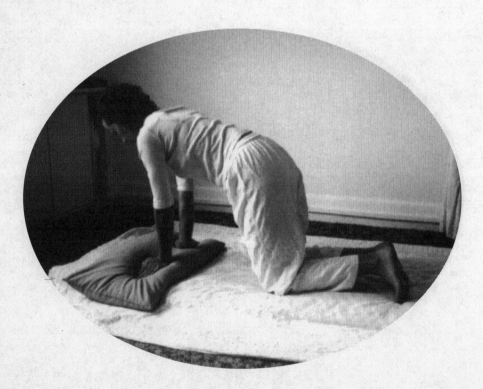

Figure 5.4b
*The third **incorrect** position.*

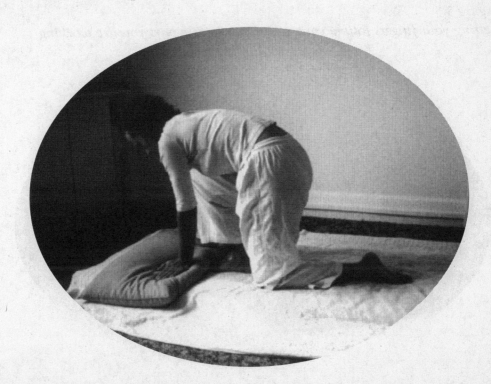

The two basic Shiatsu techniques

The two basic techniques are palming and thumbing, which I outline and illustrate as follows.

1 Palming

In palming, you use your whole hand, not the heel of your hand, to gently but firmly apply pressure. You relax your fingers so they follow the contours of your recipient's bodily part you are working, as shown in Figure 5.5.

Figure 5.5
Letting your fingers follow your recipient's bodily part you are working.

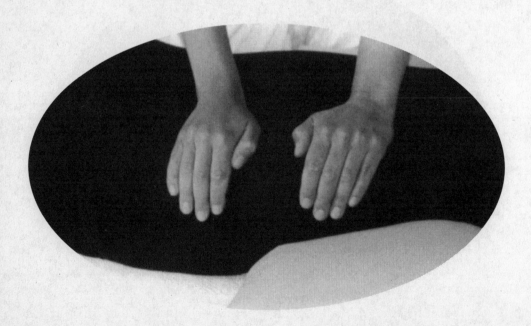

When you tonify, you slowly lean your body weight into the pressure. You lean back slowly, hold your mother hand in contact and move your other hand along your recipient's body. When you are doing this, you slowly lean forward in order to apply stationary and perpendicular pressure, as shown in Figure 5.6.

Figure 5.6
Tonifying your recipient.

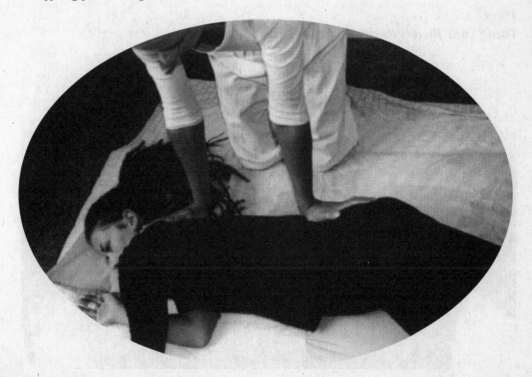

2 Thumbing

In thumbing, you use the broadness of your thumb, not the tip of it, to apply pressure that is more penetrating than the pressure you apply in palming. You use thumbing for specific tsubos (points) along a meridian. You extend your fingers to support your thumb, which you keep straight, as shown in Figure 5.7.

Figure 5.7
Using your fingers to support your thumb, which you keep straight.

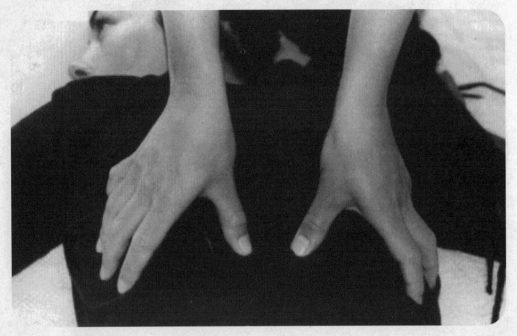

As you do in palming, you lean in, position your thumb, hold for between three and seven seconds, then ease off. You can usually press a point three times unless I specifically indicate otherwise in the directions for the following basic session.

A basic Shiatsu session for the support person to conduct

Step 1
Begin by asking your recipient to lie on her side on the futon. Use a pillow to support her knee and if necessary a "peanut" pillow to support her neck.

Step 2
Kneel beside your recipient and gently place your hand on her hip or shoulder, as shown in Figure 5.8. Slow your breathing, and focus your attention on your recipient and what she needs at this time. Begin when you feel comfortable.

Figure 5.8
Kneeling beside your recipient and gently placing your hand
on her hip or shoulder.

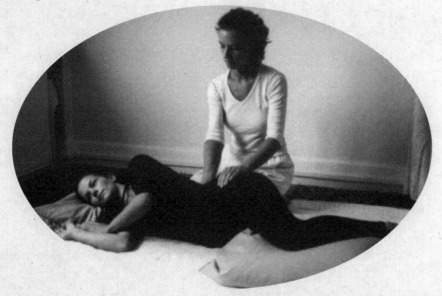

Step 3

Using both your hands, begin to work on your recipient by stretching the sides of her body, as shown in Figure 5.9. Using one of your hands, gently hold under your recipient's left shoulder; then, using your other hand, gently hold on her left hip. Straining neither yourself nor your recipient, slowly and gently stretch your arms apart. Then, in the way described, stretch the top of your recipient's spine away from her sacrum (lower-back bone), and stretch the right side of her body. Take your time, and breathe when you stretch. Each time you stretch, let yourself lean into the stretch. Ask your recipient to breathe in at the beginning of each stretch and to exhale through the stretch. Co-ordinate your breathing with hers.

Figure 5.9
Beginning to work on your recipient by stretching the sides of her body.

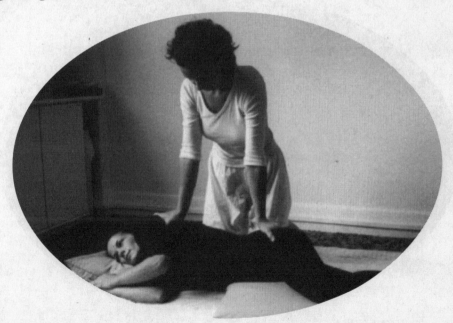

Step 4

Interlacing your hands, grasp your recipient's uppermost shoulder and slowly stretch it down towards her hips, as shown in Figure 5.10.

Figure 5.10
Grasping your recipient's uppermost shoulder and slowly stretching it down towards her hips.

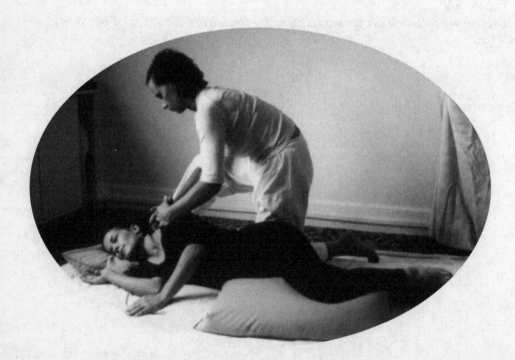

Step 5
Holding your recipient's shoulder, slowly rotate her arm in it, as shown in Figure 5.11. While you are holding her arm, support it on your chest and gently stretch it up.

Figure 5.11
Slowly rotating your recipient's arm in her shoulder.

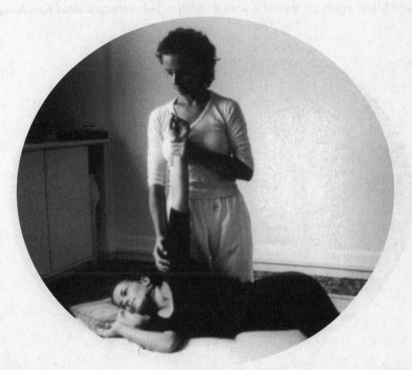

Step 6

Gently grasp your recipient's arm between your thumb and forefingers, as shown in Figure 5.12. Open and close your fingers as you move down your recipient's arm.

Figure 5.12
Gently grasping your recipient's arm between your thumb and forefingers.

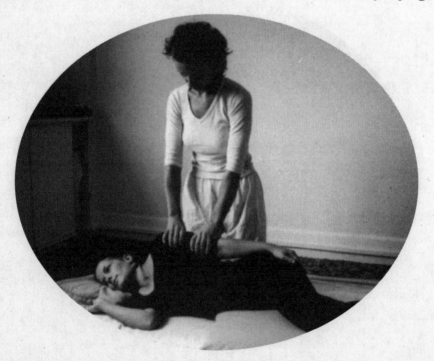

Step 7

From your recipient's shoulder to her wrist, palm her arm three times, as shown in Figure 5.13. Her arm should be lying on the side of her body, her hand resting on her hip.

Figure 5.13
Palming your recipient's arm.

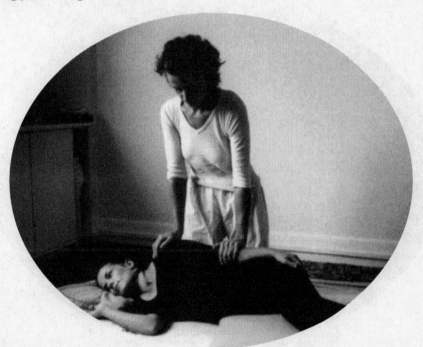

Step 8

Thumb down between the bones of your recipient's hands twice, as shown in Figure 5.14.

Figure 5.14
Thumbing down between the bones of your recipient's hands.

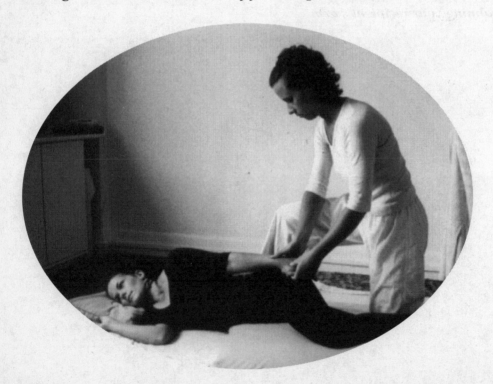

Step 9

Slowly stretch each of your recipient's fingers by grasping it between your fingers and gently sliding your fingers down it, as shown in Figure 5.15.

Figure 5.15
Slowly stretching each of your recipient's fingers.

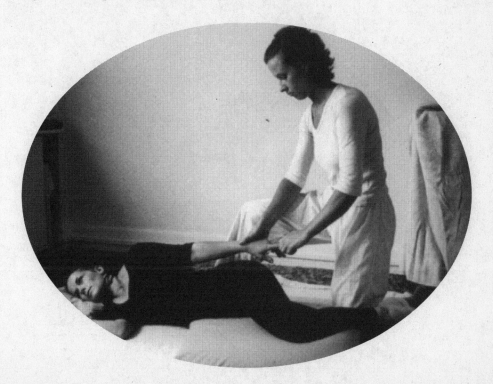

Step 10

Take your recipient's arm you have been working on and place it at her side.

Step 11

Kneeling at your recipient's back and visualising yourself as a cat, palm down her back, as shown in Figure 5.16.

Figure 5.16
Palming down your recipient's back.

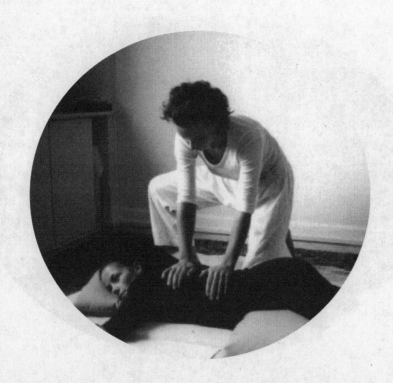

Step 12

Thumb under your recipient's scapula (shoulderblade) twice, as shown in Figure 5.17, then thumb the scapula's outer edge twice.

Figure 5.17
Thumbing under your recipient's scapula.

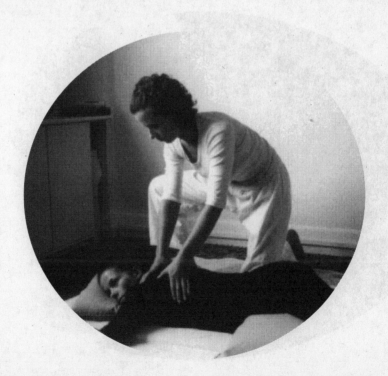

Step 13

Thumb along the area between your recipient's spine and ribs, as shown in Figure 5.18.

Figure 5.18
Thumbing along the area between your recipient's spine and ribs.

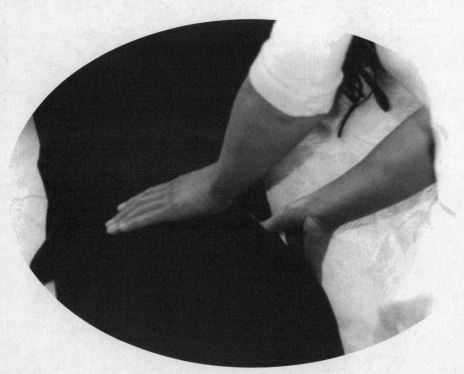

Step 14

Resting your mother hand on either your recipient's hips or the top of her back, palm down her back, as shown in Figure 5.19.

Figure 5.19
Palming down your recipient's back.

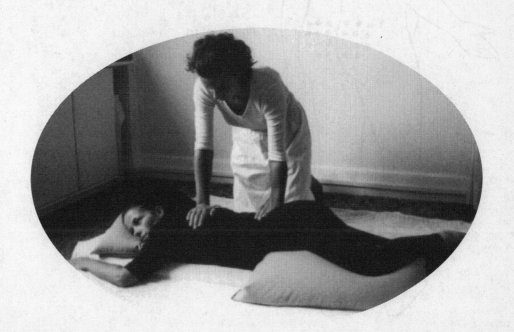

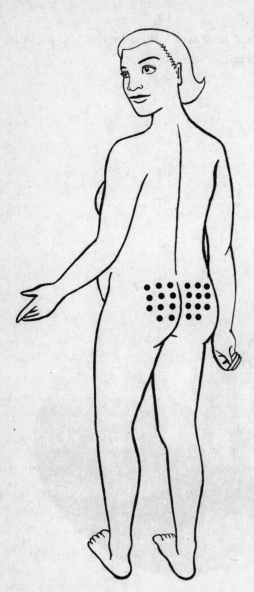

Step 15

Thumb down the middle of your recipient's sacrum (lower-back bone) three times. The sacral points are illustrated in Figure 5.20.

Figure 5.20
The sacral points.

Step 16

Using your palm or fist, lean into your recipient's hip area, as shown in Figure 5.21. Spend as much time working on this area as your recipient requires, because this technique can produce a lot of relief in the pregnant woman's hip area, where she carries most of the baby's weight.

Figure 5.21
Leaning into your recipient's hip area.

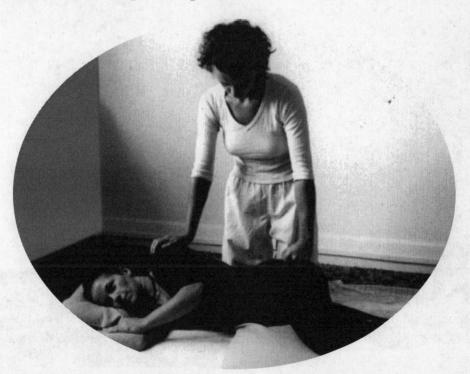

Step 17

Place your mother hand on your recipient's hip. Then, using your other hand, start from your recipient's hip and work down her leg by gently palming the outside of it (the outside-leg seam line of her trousers) three times, as shown in Figure 5.22.

Figure 5.22
Working down your recipient's leg by gently palming the outside of it.

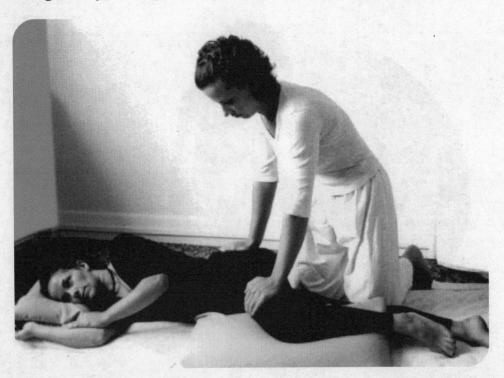

Step 18

Palm along the inside of your recipient's underneath leg (the inside-leg seam line of her trousers) twice, as shown in Figure 5.23.

Figure 5.23
Palming along the inside of your recipient's underneath leg.

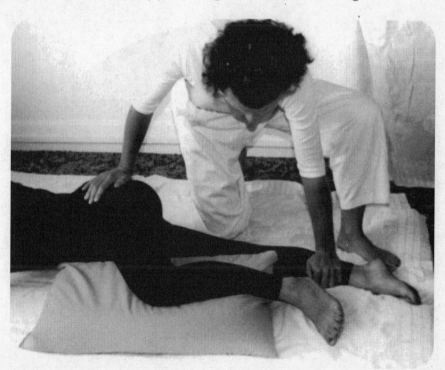

Step 19

Thumb around your recipient's heel, which is another area that is placed under a lot of strain during pregnancy. Using both your hands, stretch your recipient's foot out between your hands, both sideways and lengthwise, as shown in Figure 5.24.

Figure 5.24
Stretching your recipient's foot out between your hands,
both sideways and lengthwise.

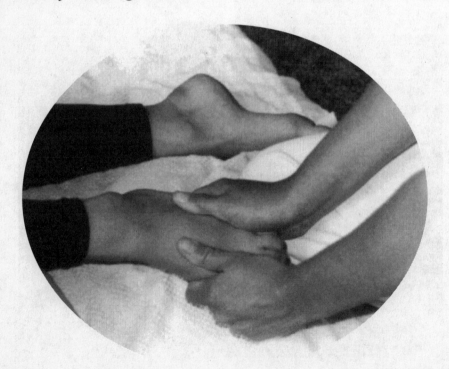

Repeat steps 1 to 19 on the other side of your recipient's body. It takes about twenty minutes to complete each nineteen-step sequence for each side. Then continue your therapy by completing steps 20 to 30 as follows.

Step 20
Ask your recipient to lie on her back. Place a pillow under her knees in order to support her knees and legs.

Step 21
If your recipient has long hair, slowly move it up and out of the way. Then, using both your hands through to your fingertips, stroke from the base of her skull to the top of her skull three times. Always move from the base to the top of the skull, not the other way around.

Step 22

Your thumbs flattened, gently stroke from the top of your recipient's skull to the point Yingtan between her eyebrows, as shown in Figure 5.25. Stroke by following one thumb after the other, and complete the step twenty times.

Figure 5.25
Gently stroking from the top of your recipient's skull
to the point Yingtan between her eyebrows.

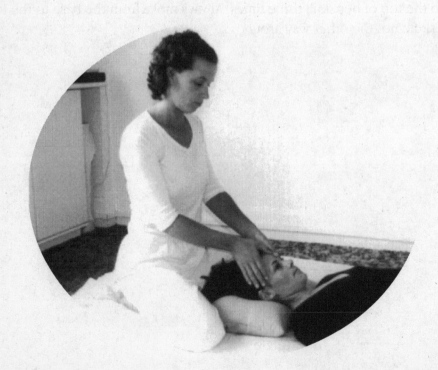

Step 23

Resting your thumbs above your recipient's nose, where her eyebrows begin, stroke and gently stretch her forehead to her temples, as shown in Figure 5.26. Complete the step twenty times.

Figure 5.26
Stroking and gently stretching your recipient's forehead to her temples.

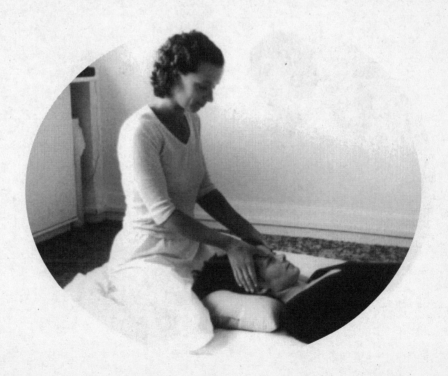

Step 24

Placing your fingertips on the sides of your recipient's head, massage all over her head in a circular motion, as shown in Figure 5.27. Start at the sides of her head, move to the centre, then move back to the sides. Do not rush when you are using this technique, because it is calming and most recipients thoroughly enjoy it.

Figure 5.27
Massaging all over your recipient's head in a circular motion.

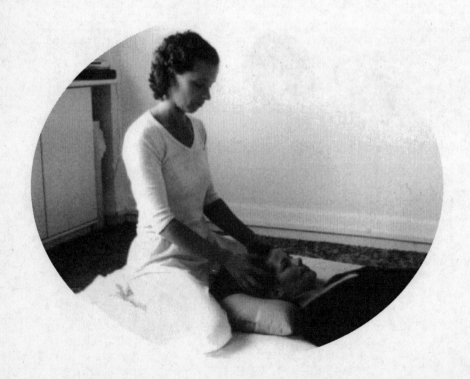

Step 25

Move to your recipient's side. Then, supporting her arm at her shoulder joint, lift the arm by the wrist and gently rotate the shoulder at its joint, as shown in Figure 5.28.

Figure 5.28
Gently rotating your recipient's shoulder at its joint.

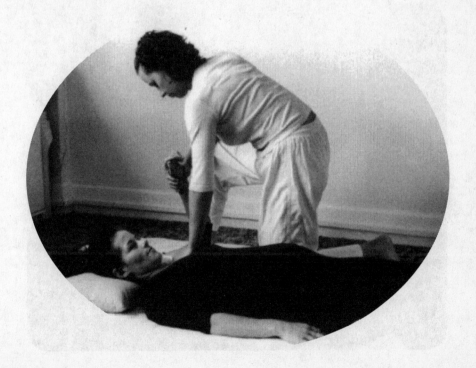

Step 26

Lay your recipient's arm at a right angle to her head. Then palm from the top of her arm to her wrist three times, as shown in Figure 5.29. Repeat the step on the opposite side of your recipient's body.

Figure 5.29
Palming from the top of your recipient's arm to her wrist.

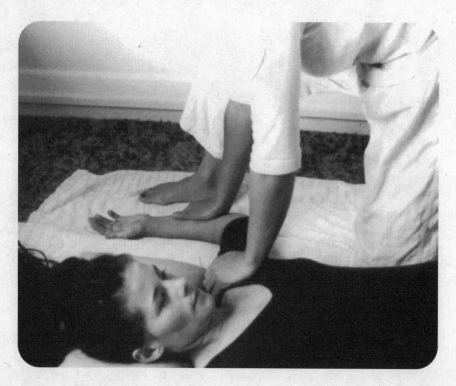

Step 27

Trying to maintain contact with your recipient's body as you move down, slowly move yourself to her feet. Grasp one of her ankles and gently stretch it towards your Hara, as shown in Figure 5.30a.

Figure 5.30a
Gently stretching your recipient's ankle towards your Hara.

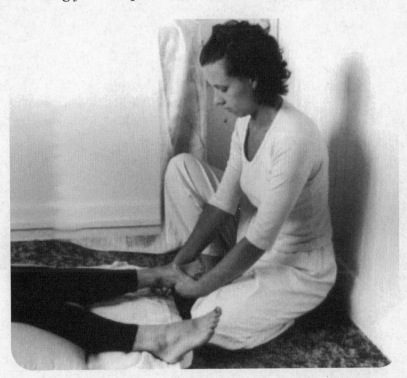

Then turn your recipient's leg inwards and stretch it. Straighten her leg, then palm from the top of it to her foot twice, as shown in Figure 5.30b. Repeat the step for your recipient's other leg.

Figure 5.30b
Palming from the top of your recipient's leg to her foot.

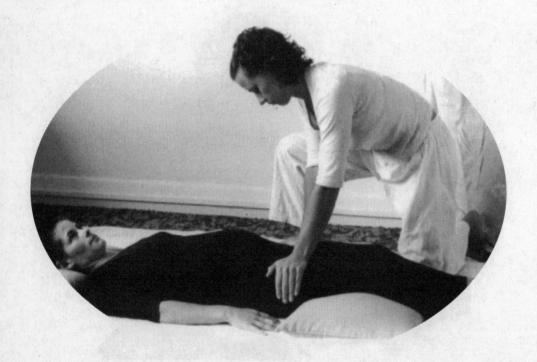

Step 28

Rotate one of your recipient's ankle joints. Then, using both your hands, stretch and knead her foot, as shown in Figure 5.31. Repeat the step for your recipient's other ankle and foot. Working with your recipient's feet helps you to keep her "grounded".

Figure 5.31
Stretching and kneading your recipient's foot.

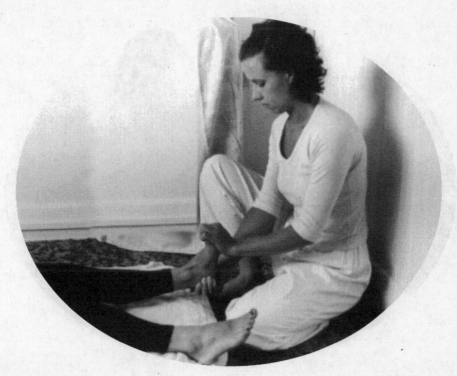

Step 29

Kneel beside your recipient. Then lay your hands on her abdomen, as shown in Figure 5.32.

Figure 5.32
Laying your hands on your recipient's abdomen.

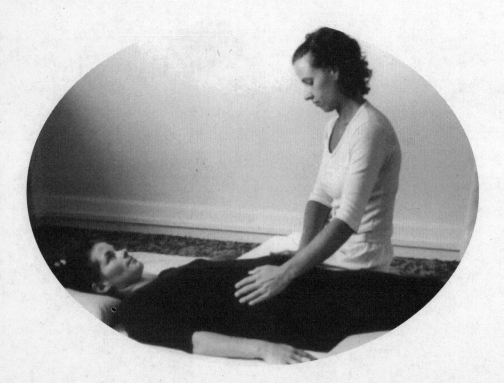

Step 30

Slowly and gently stroke around one side of your recipient's abdomen, as shown in Figure 5.33. Then, very gently and non-intrusively, stroke up to her navel and down the other side of her abdomen. Continue stroking until you have worked her whole abdomen.

Figure 5.33
Slowly and gently stroking around your recipient's abdomen.

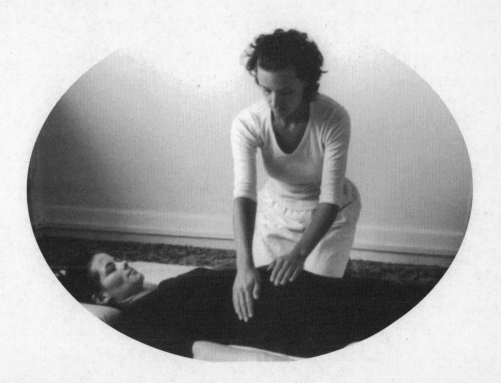

Step 31

Finish by gently resting one of your hands on your recipient's abdomen. When you feel your breathing becoming less slow and returning to normal, slowly disengage from your recipient. Let her rise when she is ready.

6
Conditions that might occur during pregnancy

In this chapter, I alphabetically list and discuss the following conditions that can occur during pregnancy: abdominal pain, adverse uprising of foetal energy, dysuria, eclampsia gravidarum, intractable cough, involuntary spasm of the lower limbs, miscarriage, morning sickness, oedema and vaginal bleeding. I outline what the conditions' causes, symptoms and treatments are according to practitioners of Traditional Chinese Medicine, and illustrate the points used for treating each condition. When appropriate, I suggest a treatment for the Shiatsu recipient's support person to apply.

Abdominal pain during pregnancy

Causes

For the pregnant woman, abdominal pain can be caused by

1   Cold Invasion
2   Qi and Blood Deficiency
3   Qi Stagnation
4   Food Stagnation.

Following are the symptoms and treatments for each of the four causes and the suggested points for the support person to use.

1   Cold Invasion

Symptoms

Your recipient might feel cold internally, might have a puffy face and might produce loose stools (faeces). Her pulse will be deep and wiry, and her tongue will be pale and have a thin, white, sticky coating.

Treatment

- Cold Invasion responds well to herbal and dietary therapy. Suggest your recipient drink small amounts of either ginger tea or tarragon tea, and that she both keep warm and refrain from eating either cold or raw foods.
- Do not use moxa on your recipient's stomach if she is in the first trimester. Personally, I prefer not to use moxa for Cold Invasion, because it can distress the foetus.

2 Qi and Blood Deficiency

Symptoms

Your recipient will have a dragging pain over her lumbar and abdominal area as well as downward pressure. She might be listless, have a poor appetite, have a pale complexion, feel dizzy and have heart palpitations. Her tongue might be pale and have a whitish coating, and her pulse might be either weak and thready or large and hollow.

Treatment

Qi and Blood Deficiency also responds well to herbal and dietary therapy. Suggest your recipient both have plenty of rest and eat warm, nourishing foods such as a soup made from bones and vegetables, which she will also digest easily. Also suggest she purchase Bhu Zhong Yi Qi Wan, a formula that is available in pill form.

3 Qi Stagnation

Symptoms

Your recipient will have congestion and pain in either her abdomen and upper abdomen or under her ribs. She might have a feeling of distension in her abdomen, her intestines might be borborygmic (have gas rumblings in them), and she might be depressed and irritable. She might also be excessively thirsty, have a bitter taste in her mouth, have concentrated urine and be constipated. Her tongue will have a thin, sticky coating, and her pulse will be wiry.

Treatment

- Suggest your recipient both place a warm hot-water bottle on her stomach and drink at least six cups of warm water a day.

- Suggest she reduce her intake of coffee and tea, because they have a diuretic effect.
- For dietary suggestions, please refer to "Chapter 9: Lifestyle and dietary therapy".

4 Food Stagnation

Symptoms
Your recipient might feel bloated or full in her stomach, regurgitate her food, have a reduced appetite and have undigested food in her faeces. Her tongue might have a sticky, white coating.

Treatment
- Suggest your recipient have dietary therapy.
- Suggest she drink the useful herbal formula Po Chai with warm water.

A suggested treatment for the support person to apply
- Use the two points PC6 and BL17.
- Gently palm pressure to the point CV12.

Figure 6.1 The points used for treating abdominal pain during pregnancy.

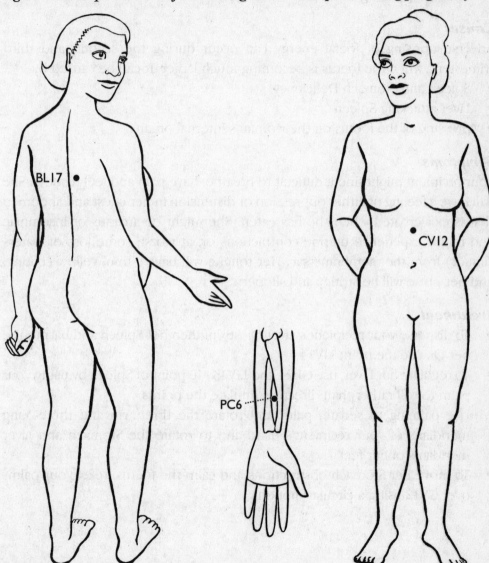

Adverse uprising of foetal energy

Causes
Adverse uprising of foetal energy can occur during the second and third trimesters, when the foetus is becoming much larger. It can be caused by
- Spleen and Stomach Deficiency
- Liver attacking Spleen
- pressing of the foetus on the woman's internal organs.

Symptoms
Your recipient might find it difficult to breathe, have pain and feel restless. She will have a feeling of either oppression or distension in her chest and abdomen that is exacerbated when she has eaten. She might be anxious or insomniac and might experience uterine contractions or, at worst, some loss of waters (liquor) from the membrane sac. Her tongue will have a thin, yellow coating, and her pulse will be stringy and slippery.

Treatment
- To disperse your recipient's Liver Qi, strengthen her Spleen and harmonise her Qi, use the point LIV14.
- To regulate her Liver, use GB24 and LIV13 Mu point of Spleen by using your palm to roll rather than directly stimulate the points.
- Use palming to sedate, palm and rotate the three Yin and three Yang meridians of your recipient's hand and to rotate the Stomach and Liver meridians of her feet.
- To move her Stomach obstructions and calm the foetus, relax your palms over CV12 using a circular motion.

***A suggested treatment for the support
person to apply***

- To help descend your recipient's Qi, use firm pressure to work her feet, then stretch and knead them. Finally, hold them for about five minutes.
- In a circular motion, gently massage to the point CV12, then hold for about five minutes.

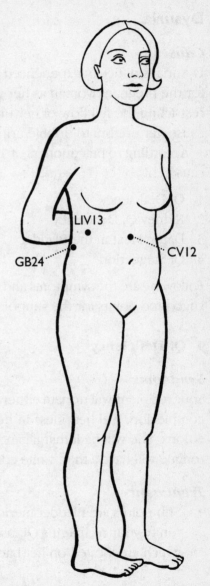

*Figure 6.2 The points used for treating
adverse uprising of foetal energy.*

Dysuria

Causes

Dysuria is difficulty experienced in fully discharging urine. It is to be expected for the pregnant woman as her growing baby presses on her bladder, thereby restricting the full flow of her urine. Her baby's weight and pressure can also cause her urethra to dribble urine when she coughs and sneezes.

According to practitioners of Traditional Chinese Medicine, dysuria is usually caused by

1 Qi Deficiency
2 Kidney Qi Deficiency
3 Damp Heat in the Bladder
4 Qi Stagnation.

Following are the symptoms and treatments for each of the four causes and the suggested points for the support person to use.

1 Qi Deficiency

Symptoms

Your recipient will urinate either scantily or infrequently and might have a pale complexion, feel heaviness in her head, feel dizzy and even have heart palpitations. She will be lethargic and have some lower-abdominal distension. Her tongue will have a thin, white coating, and her pulse will be weak and slippery.

Treatment

- Shu points are Bladder-meridian points associated with specific organs. To tonify your recipient's Qi, use the Shu points BL13, BL20, BL23 and BL28, which are located on her back.

- Suggest she both elevate her legs as much as possible and sit rather than stand for long periods.
- Inform her that if she does what you suggest, the baby will not weigh on her bladder as much.

2 Kidney Qi Deficiency

Symptoms

Your recipient will urinate either scantily or infrequently and might have oedema (fluid retention) in her face and body. She will have both lethargy and aching in her lower limbs and lower-back area, and might have abdominal distension. She will produce watery stools and have an aversion to coldness. Her tongue will be pale and have a thin, white coating, and her pulse will be either deepish and possibly slow or slippery and weak.

Treatment

- To warm your recipient's Kidney Yang, use the points BL23, KID3 and KID7.
- To transform her Qi and Fluids, use BL22 and BL28.

3 Damp Heat in the Bladder

Symptoms

Your recipient's symptoms might be similar to those of cystitis. Her urination time might be short, her urine might be concentrated and she might feel heat internally while she is urinating. She might have either a reddish or a flushed complexion, feel heaviness in her head and have a bitter taste in her mouth. Her stools might be irregular: either they will be watery or she will be constipated. Her tongue will be reddish and have a thin, greasy, yellow coating, and her pulse will be rapid.

Treatment

- To remove your recipient's Heat and Damp and clear the Fire in her Lower Jiao, use the point LIV2.
- To stimulate her Kidney Yin, use KID9.
- To regulate her Lower Jiao, use SP9 carefully, as well as BL28 and BL32.
- Suggest she drink a tea made from dried-out corn silk (the hair-like "silk" around the cob) three times a day until her symptoms cease.

4 Qi Stagnation

Symptoms

Your recipient might have this condition from the beginning to the end of her pregnancy. She might have lower-abdominal distension and find it difficult to urinate. She might feel oppressed in her chest, suffer heartburn, be anxious and depressed and find it difficult to lie in a stretched position. Her tongue will be tooth marked and swollen and have a thin, sticky coating, and her pulse will be deep and wiry.

Treatment

Qi Stagnation responds well to dietary and lifestyle therapy.

- To move your recipient's Qi, use the point SP9 cautiously.
- To regulate her Qi circulation, use LIV3.
- To treat her dysuria in general, use SP7.
- To regulate her Lower Jiao, use BL32 and BL38.

A suggested treatment for the support person to apply

- Palm your recipient's back and sacrum (lower-back bone).
- Use the point KID3.

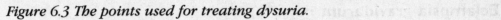

Figure 6.3 The points used for treating dysuria.

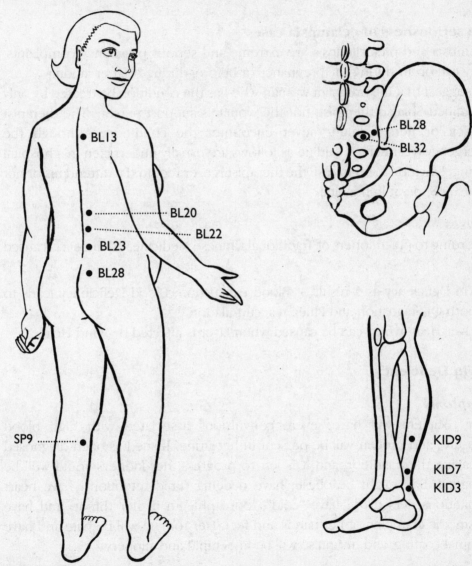

Eclampsia gravidarum

The seriousness of eclampsia cases

Eclampsia and pre-eclampsia are extreme and serious pregnancy complaints. They can occur during the pregnancy or before, during or after labour.

I suggest that the pregnant woman who has the condition be treated by only a qualified Shiatsu therapist, not the woman's support person. The therapist himself or herself might never encounter the condition. Although the emergency treatments I outline as follows are usually undertaken in a hospital setting, I include them in case the therapist is ever required to attend his or her Shiatsu recipient in hospital.

Causes

According to practitioners of Traditional Chinese Medicine, eclampsia is caused by

1 Yin Deficiency as a result of Blood exhaustion; Blood Deficiency leads to both Qi Stagnation and Phlegm accumulation
2 Liver Heat, which can be caused when Liver is affected by Wind Heat.

1 Yin Deficiency

Symptoms

Your recipient will have severe convulsions associated with high blood pressure, and protein will be present in her urine. If she has been diagnosed as having the condition and it is left to progress, her kidneys could well be damaged. She might be obese; have oedema (fluid retention); have heart palpitations; feel dizzy; have "cold", loose phlegm in her throat; and have spasmodic cramping of her hands and feet. Her tongue will be pale and have minimal coating, and her pulse will be fine, rapid and slippery.

Treatment

- To nourish your recipient's Blood, use the points BL15, BL17, BL20, BL38 and SP8.
- To move her Qi, use BL15, BL18, CV6, CV17, GB34 and ST36.
- To move her Phlegm, use BL22, LU9, SP9 and ST40.

2 Liver Heat

Symptoms

Sometimes, pregnant women who have eclampsia have symptoms of both Liver Heat and Wind Heat. In this case, your recipient will have a reddish complexion, have blurred vision, feel dizzy, be anxious and have heart palpitations. She might produce dry stools, have tidal fever (erratic bouts of high temperature and normal temperature during the day), faint and have cramping or twitching. Her tongue will be red and have a thin, dry, yellow coating, and her pulse will be rapid and wiry.

Treatment

- To improve your recipient's Kidney Yin, use the point KID3.
- To improve her Blood and reduce her Liver Heat, use BL17, BL20, BL23 and KID3.
- To reduce her Liver Heat, use LIV2.
- To dispel her Wind, use GB20 and GB37 Luo point of Liver.

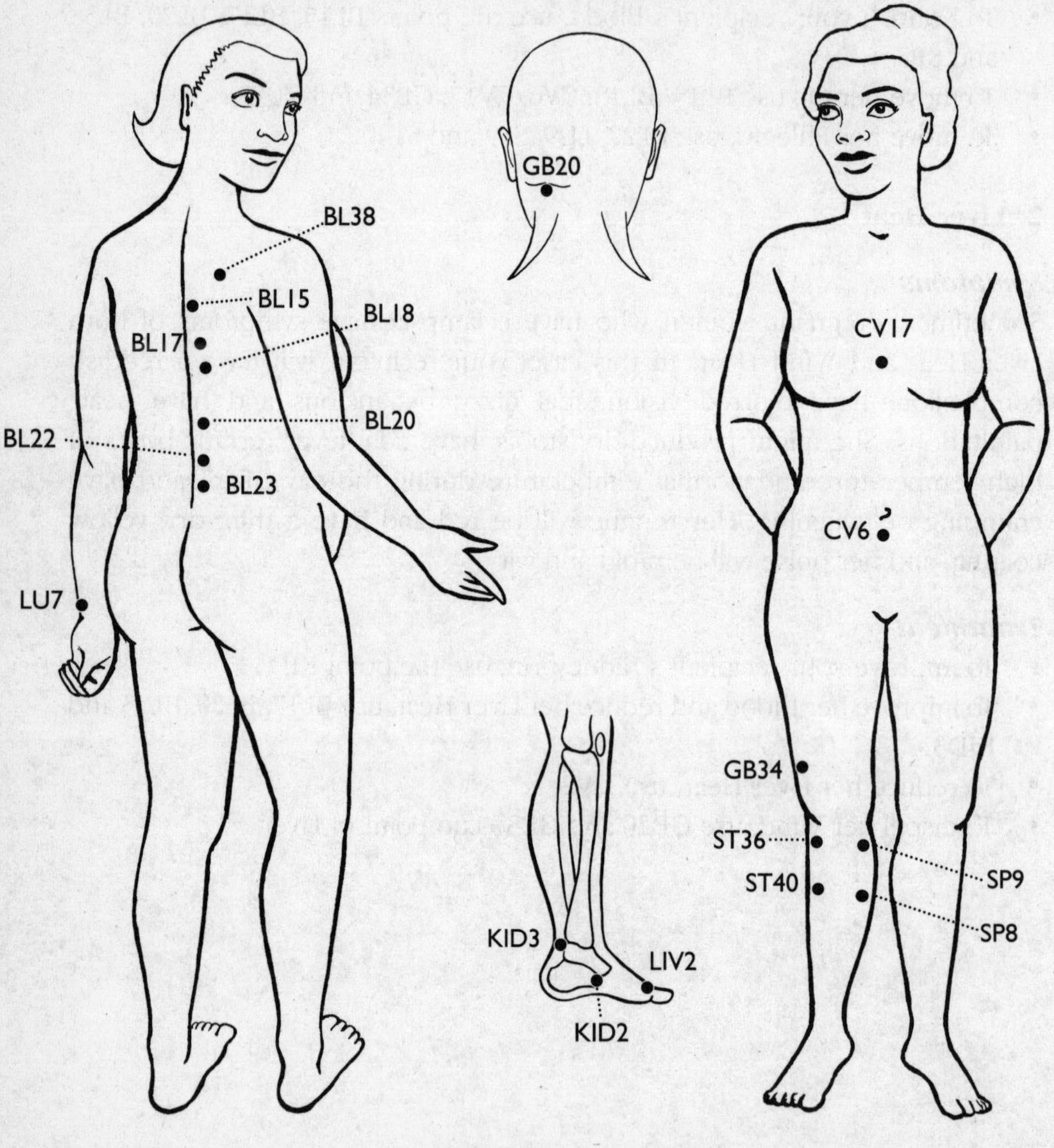

Figure 6.4 The points used for treating eclampsia gravidarum.

BL38
BL15
BL18
BL17
BL22
BL20
BL23
LU7

GB20

CV17
CV6

GB34
ST36
ST40
SP9
SP8

KID3
LIV2
KID2

Intractable cough

Causes

An intractable cough is a persistent cough that is not easily dealt with. According to practitioners of Traditional Chinese Medicine, it is caused by Heat Deficiency as a result of Lung and Kidney Yin Deficiency. Alternatively, it can be caused when the body is invaded by exogenous Wind or Cold, that is, Wind or Cold that originates outside the body.

Symptoms

Having an intractable cough can be very distressing for the pregnant woman. She might be anxious, and both her palms and the soles of her feet might feel hot. She might have an erratic fever, be sweaty at night, produce blood-stained sputum, feel dizzy, have a dry throat, have flushed cheeks, be lethargic and lose weight. Her tongue will be dry and have a thin and yellow or minimal coating, and her pulse will be thready, rapid and slippery.

Treatment

Treatment of your recipient's intractable cough involves nourishing her Yin, moistening her Lung, stopping her cough and calming the foetus.

- To release her chest and regulate her lungs, use the point CV17.
- To regulate her lungs, slowly apply sustained pressure to BL13.
- To regulate her Conception Vessel, sedate LU7.
- To regulate and calm her lungs, use LU9.
- To move her stagnant Liver Qi, use LIV13.
- Work LU5, BL23 and BL52 using your elbow or thumb.
- Calm her chest by using Jin Shin Do on LU1 and supporting ribcage pressure using CV17.
- To clear her Heat, use SP3.

- To restore her collapsed Yin and calm the foetus, use KID3 by either using Jin Shin Do or tonifying by way of frequently applying pressure for a short time.

A suggested treatment for the support person to apply
- Hold your palm on the point CV17 for about five minutes.
- Palm the Bladder meridian of your recipient's back.
- Firmly stroke LU7 towards her head.

Figure 6.5 The points for treating intractable cough.

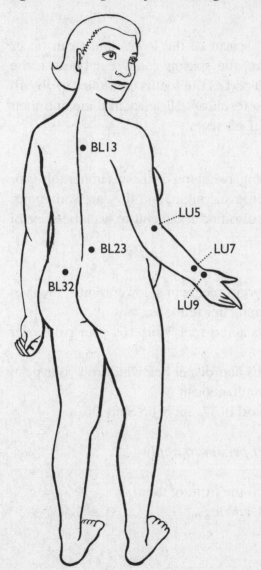
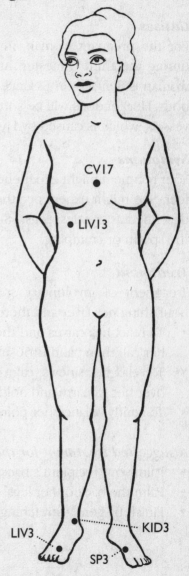

Involuntary spasm of the lower limbs

Causes

For the pregnant woman, involuntary spasm of the lower limbs can occur during the third trimester. At this time, the spasms can occur because the woman is deficient in Essence and/or Blood as the foetus continues to absorb both. Her tendons will be softened as a result of deficiency in them and their vessels, which is caused by Liver Blood Deficiency.

Symptoms

Your recipient might experience cramping, twitching or spasms in her calves or feet. She might experience these symptoms at night, and they are sometimes described as "restless legs". She might also find it difficult to walk because of the spasm or cramping.

Treatment

Treatment of involuntary spasm of your recipient's lower limbs involves nourishing her Liver and therefore calming her tendons.

- To relax her calves and their sinews and dispel Wind, roll your palm over her calf then palm BL56 and BL57.
- To relax her sinews, calm the foetus and dispel her Wind, roll your palm over her forearm and hold BL40 simultaneously.
- To gently balance her points BL40 and BL57, apply Jin Shin Do.

A suggested treatment for the support person to apply

- Palm your recipient's back.
- Palm the back of her legs, then palm the front of them.
- Finish by gently stretching her back and legs.

Figure 6.6
The points used for treating involuntary spasm of the lower limbs.

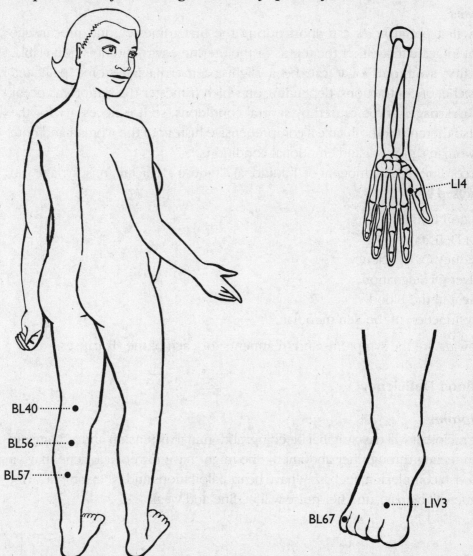

Miscarriage

Causes

Many first pregnancies can abort during the first trimester, and miscarriage might indicate that either the foetus or the uterine environment is non-viable. The first symptoms of it can be a slight haemorrhaging, some pain and backache, or contractions, depending on which trimester the symptoms occur in. Miscarriage can be caused by several conditions, so it is necessary for the Shiatsu therapist to both take a comprehensive history of the woman and note the woman's physical and emotional condition.

According to practitioners of Traditional Chinese Medicine, miscarriage can be caused by

1 Blood Deficiency
2 Qi Deficiency
3 Kidney Qi Deficiency
4 Liver Qi Stagnation
5 Heat in the Blood
6 dysfunction of the Ren meridian.

Following are the symptoms and treatments for each of the six causes.

1 Blood Deficiency

Symptoms

Your recipient will have vaginal bleeding, abdominal distension and a dragging-down feeling through her abdomen. She might have lower-back ache, have a yellowish complexion, feel dizzy, have heart palpitations and be insomniac. Her tongue will be pale, and her pulse will be fine and weak.

Treatment

- To stimulate your recipient's Qi and Blood, use the points CV4 and CV6.
- To stimulate her Blood circulation, use BL17.
- To strengthen her Blood, use BL20.
- To regulate her Qi, use BL23.
- To build her Blood, use moxa.

2 Qi Deficiency

Symptoms

Your recipient will have lower-back ache, have weak legs and knees, have tinnitus (ringing in the ears) and feel dizzy. She will have either frequent bleeding or a discharge of watery, yellow fluid. She might urinate frequently and copiously, and her sleep will be disturbed by her need to urinate. Her tongue will be pale, and her pulse will be weak in the Kidney position.

Treatment

- To regulate your recipient's Kidney Qi, tonify using the point BL23 and use Yuan Qi and GV4.
- Use moxa on BL28 and tonify CV4.

3 Kidney Qi Deficiency

Symptoms

Your recipient will have lower-back ache, have weak legs and knees, have tinnitus and feel dizzy. She might urinate frequently and copiously, and her sleep might be disturbed because she has to urinate frequently. Her tongue will be pale, and the Kidney position of her pulse will be weak.

Treatment

- To regulate your recipient's Kidney Qi, tonify using the point BL23 and tonify Yuan Qi and GV4.
- Use moxa from BL28 to GV4.

4 Liver Qi Stagnation

Symptoms

Your recipient's Liver Qi might stagnate during the second trimester, whereby she will experience foetal disturbance and have abdominal pain. She might also vomit, regurgitate acid, burp, feel oppression in her chest and have pain in her ribs. Her tongue will have a thick, greasy coating, and her pulse will be wiry and slippery.

Treatment

- To circulate your recipient's Qi and disperse her stagnant Liver Qi, use the point BL15.
- To tonify her Liver Qi, use BL18.
- To regulate her Spleen Qi and Blood, use BL20.
- To move her Liver Qi, use LIV2.
- To regulate her Qi, use TW3.
- To remove her Liver Qi stagnation, use TW6.

5 Heat in the Blood

Symptoms

Your recipient will have a vaginal discharge of blood that can range from light red to bright red. Her urine will be dark and scanty, and she might be constipated. Her face will be flushed, and she will be irritable. She might be excessively thirsty, and her mouth and throat might be dry. Her tongue will be

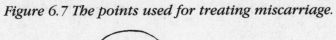

Figure 6.7 The points used for treating miscarriage.

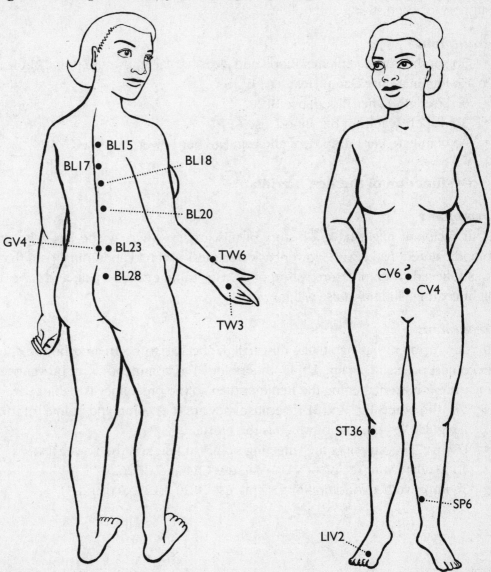

red and have a dry, yellow coating, and her pulse will be rapid as well as fine or slippery, or even strong and hollow.

Treatment
- To soothe your recipient's Blood and clear her Heat, use the point BL15.
- To eliminate her Damp Heat, use BL18.
- To strengthen her Blood, use BL20.
- To dispel Heat from her Blood, use SP10.
- To eliminate her Damp Heat and regulate her Lower Jiao, use CV3.

6 Dysfunction of the Ren meridian

Symptoms
Your recipient might have a history of miscarriage whereby she lost a lot of blood, fainted, had leg and lower-back weakness and had abdominal pain that was relieved when pressure was applied. Her tongue will be pale and have a light coating, and her pulse will be weak.

Treatment
If your recipient has habitually miscarried, she has to be treated before she becomes pregnant again. Using the points I recommend is a preventive measure for strengthening the Ren meridian so the pregnancy is viable.
- Use the points LU7 and SP4, because they are the "command points" of the Irregular Vessels, one of which is the uterus.
- Use CV7, because it is the "meeting point" of Ren and the Lower Jiao.
- To regulate your recipient's Dai Mai, use CV4 and GB26.
- To improve her condition in general, use BL20, BL23, SP6 and ST36.

Morning sickness

Causes

In the pregnant woman, the uterine collaterals – the meridians that run through the uterus – are connected to her stomach opening, so she might suffer morning sickness that can be caused by

1   Spleen and Stomach Deficiency, which leads to disharmony of the descending mechanism
2   Liver attacking Spleen, or Rebellious Qi, whereby the woman's emotional issues cause Qi to rise, or "rebel".

Symptoms

During the first trimester, the woman might feel dizzy, be nauseous and vomit. Although all three symptoms might spontaneously disappear by the advent of the second trimester, they can continue during it. If the woman's vomiting is prolonged and she is unable to eat, her Qi and Blood might become deficient and the foetus's development thereby impaired.

Following are the symptoms and treatments for each of the two causes and the suggested points for the support person to use.

1 Spleen and Stomach Deficiency

Symptoms

Your recipient will be weak in general, be nauseous, vomit and be lethargic. Her tongue will be pale and have a white coating, and her pulse will be either moderate or slippery.

Treatment

- To strengthen your recipient's Spleen and harmonise her Stomach, use palming.
- To calm her Rebellious Qi and prevent her from vomiting, apply Jin Shin Do to her middle and upper abdomen.
- Use palming to push and wipe the three Yin meridians of both sides of her head.
- To quell her feeling of sickness, use the point PC6.
- To calm her Qi, use CV12.
- To move her Phlegm and/or Damp, use ST40.
- To direct her Rebellious Qi downwards, use CV22.

2 Liver attacking Spleen

Symptoms

Your recipient's vomit will be watery and either sour or bitter. She will sigh, have a feeling of fullness in her head and have a feeling of oppression in her chest and hypochondrium – the lateral part of the abdomen, beneath the lower ribs. Her tongue will be reddish and have a slight, yellow coating, and her pulse will be stringy and slippery.

Treatment

- To disperse your recipient's Liver Qi, harmonise her Stomach and depress her Rebellious Qi, use palming to gently roll her middle to upper abdomen. Do not press hard: move towards a Jin Shin Do touch rather than a strong, rolling movement.
- To move her Liver Qi, use the point LIV14.
- To regulate her Liver, use GB24.
- Use the LIV13 Mu point of Spleen.
- To help move her Stomach obstruction, gently palm CV12.

Figure 6.8 The points used for treating morning sickness.

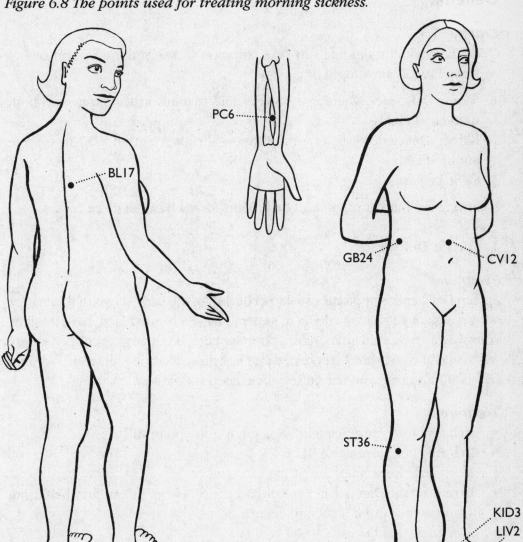

Oedema

Causes

Oedema, or fluid retention, can be a common problem during warm or hot weather. It is usually caused by

1 Spleen Deficiency, whereby the Spleen fails to transform and transport both Blood and Fluids
2 Kidney Deficiency, whereby the Kidneys are deficient and fail to excrete impure Fluids
3 Qi Stagnation.

Following are the symptoms and treatments for each of the three causes.

1 Spleen Deficiency

Symptoms

Spleen Deficiency symptoms usually occur during the early stages of pregnancy. Your recipient will have oedema in general, have a bloated face, have a sallow complexion, have cold limbs, have a poor appetite, be lethargic, produce watery stools and at worst will be depressed and feel dizzy. Her tongue will be pale and have a thin coating, and her pulse will be deep and hollow.

Treatment

- To harmonise your recipient's Spleen, use the point BL20.
- To tonify her Spleen, use BL21.
- To regulate her Damp, use SP5.
- To remove the Damp in her Lower Jiao, use SP9 – but be careful when using it, and do not use it if you are unsure.
- To regulate her Qi, use CV12.
- To regulate her Fluids, use CV9.

Figure 6.9 The points used for treating oedema.

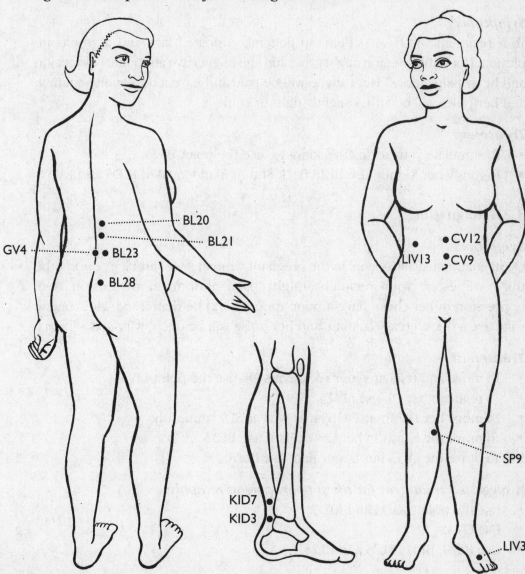

2 Kidney Deficiency

Symptoms

Your recipient will have oedema in general, a bloated face and a grey complexion. Her lumbar region might ache, and she might have abdominal distension and heart palpitations. Her tongue will be pale and have a thin, white coating, and her pulse will be either slightly tight or sunken.

Treatment

- To stimulate your recipient's kidneys, use the point BL23.
- To tonify her Kidney, use BL28 Back Shu of Bladder, GV4, KID3 and KID7.

3 Qi Stagnation

Symptoms

Qi Stagnation usually occurs in the pregnant woman's feet and legs during the third trimester. Your recipient might have abdominal distension, feel oppression in her chest, have a poor appetite and be depressed. Her tongue will have a thick, greasy coating, and her pulse will be deep, wiry and slippery.

Treatment

- To move and regulate your recipient's Qi, use the point LIV3.
- To regulate her Qi, use LIV13.
- To move her Damp, use GB34, as well as SP9 cautiously.
- To move the Fluids in her Lower Jiao, use BL22.
- To move the Qi in her Lower Jiao, use BL28.

A suggested treatment for the support person to apply

- Use the points KID3 and KID7.
- Use GV4.
- Use BL20, BL21, BL23 and BL28.

Vaginal bleeding

Causes

During pregnancy, any bleeding should be treated as important, because any loss of blood affects foetal nourishment. Vaginal bleeding can be caused by

1 Spleen Deficiency, whereby Spleen's natural ability to hold the Blood is deficient, and Qi and Yang Deficiency can also be caused as a result
2 Wind Heat, whereby an invasion of exogenous heat causes Fluids to dry up
3 Hot Blood, whereby Liver Deficiency causes excess Blood that overflows the blood vessels.

Following are the symptoms and treatments for each of the three causes and the suggested points for the support person to use.

1 Spleen Deficiency

Symptoms

Your recipient will have a sallow complexion, be lethargic, have a congested chest and produce loose stools. Her tongue will be pale and flabby and have a thin, white coating, and her pulse will be weak.

Treatment

* To tonify your recipient's Spleen, use the points BL20, BL21 and SP1.
* To increase her Yang, use GV20.
* To disperse the Damp that tends to accumulate under her clavicle and upper ribcage, gently apply pressure both across her clavicle and between her first two ribs.
* Be aware that her Spleen and Stomach points will be very sensitive to your touch.
* Consider her diet and lifestyle and make appropriate suggestions.

2 Wind Heat

Symptoms

Your recipient will feel dizzy and have a bitter taste in her mouth. She might feel hot but look cold, and her urine will be strong and concentrated. Her tongue will have a thin coating, and her pulse will be floating and rapid.

Treatment

- To dispel and strengthen your recipient's Spleen in order to hold her Blood, use the point SI11.
- To dispel her Wind, use LI1.
- To eliminate her Wind and Heat, use GB20, KID10 and LI11.
- To dispel the Heat in her Lower Jiao, use KID10.
- To dispel the Damp Heat in her Lower Jiao, use LIV8.

3 Hot Blood

Symptoms

Hot Blood can lead to miscarriage. Your recipient's blood discharge will be dark and profuse, because Liver Deficiency causes excess Blood that overflows the blood vessels. She might also have skin eruptions such as pimples and eczema. She might be irritable and have some heartburn and abdominal pain. Her tongue will have a sticky coating, and her pulse will be wiry and rapid.

Treatment

- To cool and dispel the Heat from your recipient's Blood, use the point SP10.
- To dispel the Heat in her Blood, use PC3.
- To remove the Heat from her Blood, use BL54.
- To strengthen her Blood, use BL15 and BL20.
- To strengthen her Liver, use BL18.

Figure 6.10 The points used for treating vaginal bleeding.

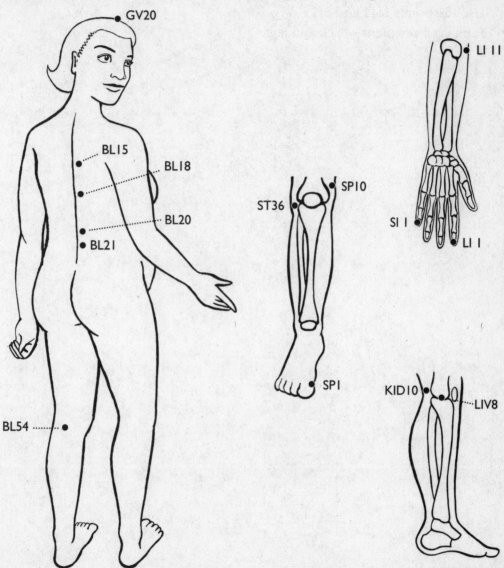

A suggested treatment for the support person to apply

- Use the points LI11 and SI1.
- Palm your recipient's back and legs.

7 Labour and birthing

The symptoms of labour

For the pregnant woman, onset of established labour is characterised by strong uterine contractions, or labour pains. Some women have pain that is similar to period cramp; others feel a wave of pain that extends from their abdomen to their lower back. Having a scattered pulse can be another indication that the woman is about to give birth.

With reference to labour pains, both their length and the intervals from one to the next vary between each woman and each pregnancy. However, the period from onset of contractions to full dilation of the cervix is usually between fifteen and twenty-four hours for first babies and eight or fewer hours for second and subsequent babies. Naturally, the fact that each woman experiences pain in her own way also has to be considered in the labour setting.

The period from full cervical dilation to the baby's birth can be between one and two hours, possibly longer, and full expulsion of the placenta can take up to one hour.

...experience of labour

...ome women, labour can have some extreme effects: vomiting, diarrhoea, incoherence as a result of the pain, and fear of the unknown. Labour is a very stressful experience for women, both physically and emotionally. Some women express the stress by screaming, crying or swearing. They are not thinking about anyone around them but are totally engrossed in their own needs – and rightly so. Anyone who is attending the birth is there to help the woman in labour *and should therefore always listen to her.*

Preparing the woman for the birth

I usually find it effective to prepare my Shiatsu recipient for her delivery about two to four weeks before the estimated date (EDD). I tell her the points that will be used and how these points will help her, and suggest positions for her to adopt during the various stages of labour.

I also give her general information and answer any questions she might have. Although the discussion might take up most of her Shiatsu-treatment time, I consider it to be anything but time lost: healing and supportive treatment involves talking as much as touching in order to maintain my recipient's confidence in me.

Your discussion time with your recipient is an opportunity for you to support her and give her information. You can discuss her needs, the pregnancy to date and the forthcoming birth.

Explaining labour pain

As the delivery date looms closer, many women experience fear of the pain they will inevitably experience, and your recipient might share her fears with you. I tell my recipient not that her birthing experience will be painless but that her pain can be managed.

I explain to my recipient that she can use breathing to "blow away the pain";

the alternative, to hold her breath, will cause her Qi to either be bl[...]
stagnate and thereby cause her pain. I tell her that breath is Qi and that b[...]
out when she feels pain will both help move Qi and reduce some of her p[...]

I always emphasise to my recipient that when she experiences strong co[...]
tractions, she will know the birth is getting closer. Because her pain might be
exaggerated as a result of the birthing position she adopts, I suggest she either
kneel on all fours, in order to take pressure off her back, or squat, in order to
both relieve her back pressure and stretch both her pelvis and her perineum.

Finding a comfortable position for labour

If your recipient asks you to attend her delivery, you should contact her
midwife before the scheduled date in order to discuss both your proposed
techniques and how your recipient and her doctor or midwife feel about your
participating.

During the labour, you should be flexible when you are treating your recipient.
I strongly suggest you let her find the position that is most comfortable for her.
As I have mentioned, some women find that kneeling on all fours helps relieve
their lower-back pain, and others prefer to squat during a contraction in order to
spread their hips and relieve some of the contraction's effects.

During the early stages of labour, your recipient might find it most comfortable to lie back in a beanbag, bend her knees and place her heels close to her
bottom. However, during the later stages, she might also find that too much
strain is placed on her lower back if she adopts this position. You will find that
most women know instinctively how to position themselves for the birth and
to find their most comfortable position.

Some women find an unusual position to be their most comfortable, in
which case their Shiatsu therapist or support person has to be flexible with
reference to the points he or she uses. If you are informing your recipient
beforehand about which points you will be required to use, ask which points

and position she prefers to use and accommodate her preferences during the labour as much as is practicable.

The support person's role during labour

Both the therapist and the support person should practise Shiatsu on themselves in order to both recognise the various amounts of pressure and understand the points' strengths and the pain associated with the points.

Mild labour is said to begin when the woman's contractions are occurring every fifteen to twenty minutes. At this stage, the best way to use the Shiatsu points is to use as many of the ones illustrated in Figure 7.1 as possible during each contraction. You should also apply heat packs to your recipient's back in order to relieve her pain between the contractions.

The Shiatsu techniques and points to use during labour

During mild labour, it is best for your recipient if she feels your pressure as a long, aching sensation. Hold the pressure for about seven seconds, then release. Repeat this technique at least three times before you move on to the next specific point.

Be aware that although the points SP6 and SP9 can be painful during labour, you should try to work them because they have a very strong ability to descend Qi. The points LIV3 and BL67 can also be very painful, so when you are working any of these points, you should listen to your recipient when she is expressing her needs.

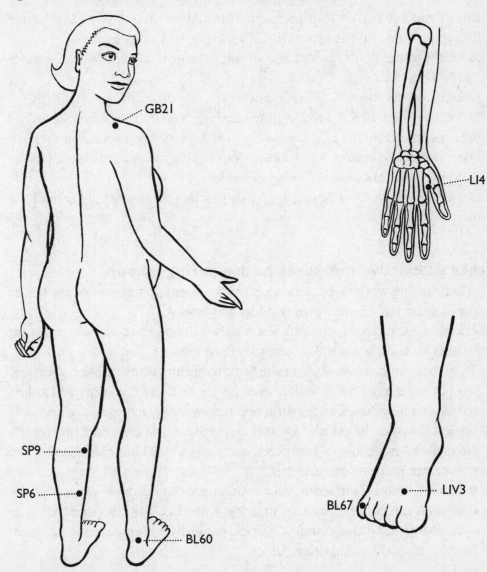

Figure 7.1 The points used for treating labour pain.

A suggested way to use Shiatsu points during labour

1 Knead and rub across your recipient's shoulders while you sedate (apply thumb pressure to) the point GB21 (see Figure 7.1 on page 127).
2 Move on to the point LI4 and use strong pressure to hold there. Consider your recipient's needs.
3 Stretch and stroke each of her hands separately, down to her fingertips.
4 Sedate the points SP6 and SP9 by firmly running your thumbs from each of her big toes up each of her legs separately, to SP9. Do not run your thumbs back down her leg. Repeat the firm rubbing from her big toe upwards at least twice.
5 Hold the point LIV3 for as long as possible.
6 Hold the point BL67 while you are either pinching or gently pulling her little toes.

Other supportive measures to use during labour

- When you are working on your recipient's Shiatsu points, do not ask her to position herself for your own comfort and ease.
- Encourage her to regularly drink warm liquids in order to both help replenish her bodily fluids and protect her from Cold Invasion.
- To aid her contractions, suggest she bring along and drink raspberry-leaf tea.
- Do not encourage her to either suck on ice or drink cold liquids. Explain to her that if she does, her contraction pain will only increase. Ice and cold liquids slow her Blood and Qi and can either slow or retard her body's circulation, especially in her pelvic area. Also, drinking cold liquids can reduce her Kidney Yang strength.
- Because labour is hard work, your recipient might become very hot. If she does, you can cool her face by applying a wet face washer (face towel) to it. However, keep suggesting she drink either room-temperature or warm liquids rather than cold ones.

Inducing labour

In my experience, it is evident that using Shiatsu techniques during labour helps to reduce labour time, to speed up contractions and to enable the woman to recover quickly after delivery. Using the points illustrated in Figure 7.1 protects both Qi and Blood.

If you wish to stimulate labour, you can choose one of the following three basic Shiatsu techniques.

1   You could strongly sedate the points BL31, BL32, LI4 and SP6.
2   You could use the points BL67, GB21, LI4 and SP6.
3   You could use the points GV1, LI4, SP6 and SP9.

If you use these points, you will regulate your recipient's Qi, move her Blood and strengthen her contractions.

Whether or not you apply moxa in order to both protect and strengthen your recipient's Kidney Yin and Kidney Yang, suggest she drink warm liquids so the same results are produced.

The points to use for inducing labour

See Figure 7.2 on page 130 for the points I mention.

- To support the induction, tonify BL32, CV4, LI4, SP6 and ST36.
- If your recipient's contractions are weak and her cervix is slow to dilate, use either LI4 and ST36 or LI4 and SP6.
- To relieve her labour pain, either use GB21, LI4, SP6, LI13, BL60 and BL67 or simply apply strong pressure to BL60 only.
- If her labour is difficult, if possible apply moxa to BL67, LI4 and SP6. Remember that using moxa both protects and strengthens Kidney Yin and Kidney Yang.
- If her labour is difficult and it is more convenient to use her ear points, stimulate the ears' Uterus and Endocrine points, as shown in Figure 7.3 on page 131.

Figure 7.2 The points used for stimulating and supporting labour, supporting induction, speeding up contractions and reducing pain.

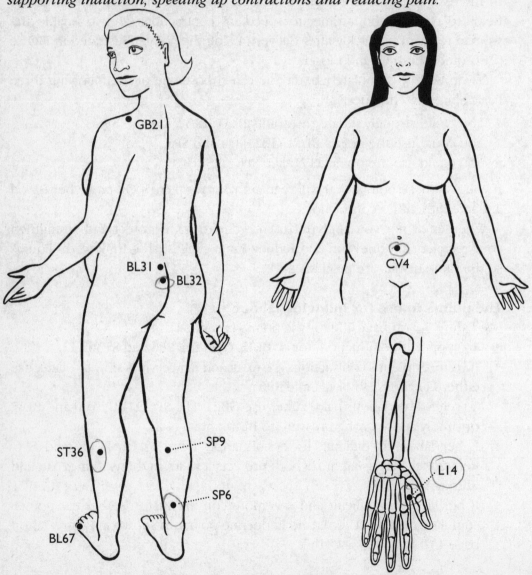

Figure 7.3 The Uterus and Endocrine ear points.

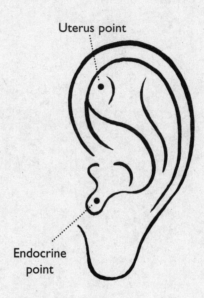

Uterus point

Endocrine
point

8
Conditions that might occur after the birth

In this chapter, I alphabetically list and discuss the following conditions that can occur after the birth: abdominal pain, arthralgia, constipation, fainting, insomnia, lactation scantiness, lochia retention, lochiorrhoea, mastitis, placenta retention, postnatal depression and urinary incontinence. I outline what the conditions' causes, symptoms and treatments are according to practitioners of Traditional Chinese Medicine, and illustrate the points used for treating each condition.

The support person should be aware that it is best for the pregnant woman if these conditions are treated by only a qualified Shiatsu therapist. If you are the support person for a pregnant woman who has any of the conditions, please consult her doctor, midwife or Shiatsu therapist.

Abdominal pain after the birth

Causes

Continuous abdominal pain after the birth can be caused by

1   Blood Stagnation, which can be related to lochia retention
2   Blood Deficiency, as a result of postnatal haemorrhaging
3   Cold Deficiency.

Following are the symptoms and treatments for each of the three causes.

1 Blood Stagnation

Symptoms

If your recipient has abdominal pain, her Blood Stagnation symptoms can be related to retention of lochia, which is the residual blood that is discharged for eight to ten days after the birth. She will have either a scanty discharge or no discharge at all. She might either vomit or have indigestion (dyspepsia), and her abdomen will be distended, possibly lumpy, and painful, especially when pressure is applied to it. Her tongue will either be slightly purple or have purple markings, and her pulse will be deep and slow.

Treatment

To alleviate your recipient's symptoms, use the points BL32, LI4, LIV3, SP6, SP10 and ST29.

Figure 8.1 The points used for treating abdominal pain after the birth.

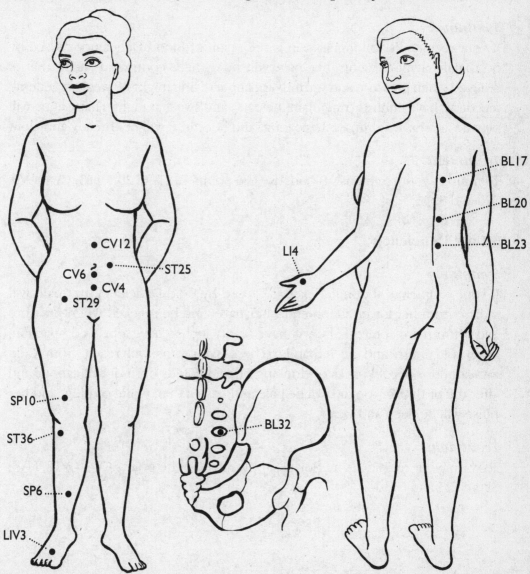

2 Blood Deficiency

Symptoms

If your recipient's abdominal pain is the result of Blood Deficiency caused by postnatal haemorrhaging, her pain will be a mild, continuous ache that is relieved when pressure and warmth are applied. She might be weak in general, feel dizzy, have tinnitus (ringing in the ears) and sweat at night. Her tongue will be pale and have a thin, white coating, and her pulse will be thready and slow.

Treatment

To nourish your recipient's Blood, use the points BL17, BL20, BL23, CV4, CV6, SP6 and ST36.

3 Cold Deficiency

Symptoms

If your recipient's abdominal pain is caused by Cold Deficiency, her pain will radiate from her lower abdomen to her navel and be relieved when pressure and warmth are applied. She will have scanty lochia, have a pale complexion, have cold limbs and be lethargic. These symptoms will result from Cold invasion, use of cold packs or drinking of cold liquids both during labour and after the birth. Her tongue will be pale and have a thin, white coating, and her pulse will be deep and weak.

Treatment

To warm your recipient's meridians, apply moxa to the points CV4, CV12, LIV3, SP6, ST25 and ST36.

Arthralgia

Causes

After the birth, arthralgia, or sinew and tendon pain, can be caused by

1 Blood and Qi Deficiency
2 Cold Wind Invasion.

Following are the symptoms and treatments for each of the two causes.

1 Blood and Qi Deficiency

Symptoms

Your recipient will have a pale, sallow complexion; be lethargic; feel dizzy; have heart palpitations; have joint pain; have numb limbs; and have localised stiffness that is alleviated when pressure is applied to the area. Her tongue will be pale red and have minimal coating, and her pulse will be thready and stringy.

Treatment

- To support your recipient's Qi, nourish her Blood and calm her tendons, apply sedation and some scraping to the point GB21.
- Sedate the points LI10 and TW5.
- Rotate and stretch her arms and legs.
- Tonify all parts of her legs.
- To stimulate her Blood and Qi, apply short, pecking pressure to her legs, and include the points KID6 and ST36.

2 Cold Wind Invasion

Symptoms

Your recipient will have joint pain, have localised stiffness, have pain that either moves or "wanders", possibly have localised numbness and swelling and be averse to the wind and/or cold. These symptoms will usually be alleviated when warmth is applied. Her tongue will be pale and have a thin, white coating, and her pulse will either be thready or be stringy and rapid.

Treatment

To nourish your recipient's Blood, expel her Wind and disperse her Cold and Dry wetness, use any or all of the following techniques.

- To dispel her Wind and Cold, tonify the point GB20 and use the point GB31.
- To dispel her Wind, use LI11 and LU5.
- To dispel her Wind and relax her sinews, use LI4.
- To relax her sinews and alleviate her pain, use GV26.
- To relax her sinews, use BL60.
- To warm her Cold, use CV4 and GV12.
- To regulate and tonify her Liver, use GB34.
- To benefit her knees, use ST35.
- Rotate and stretch her legs and arms.
- To harmonise her Conception Vessel (CV) meridian, apply Jin Shin Do.

Figure 8.2 The points used for treating arthralgia.

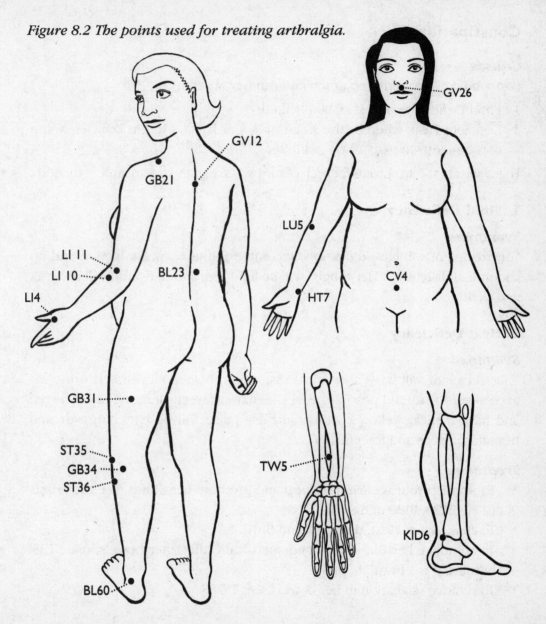

Constipation

Causes

Postnatal constipation is common and can be caused by

1 Fluid Deficiency, or loss of bodily fluids
2 Deficient Heat, whereby the strain of labour has led to Yin Deficiency and consequently to exhaustion of Fluids.

Following are the symptoms for each of the two causes and the treatment for both.

1 Fluid Deficiency

Symptoms

Your recipient will have a dry, sallow complexion; a normal appetite; and no abdominal distension. Her tongue will be light red, and her pulse will be weak and slow.

2 Heat Deficiency

Symptoms

Your recipient will have abdominal distension, have concentrated urine, be excessively thirsty and possibly be febrile (have a fever). Her tongue will be red and have a sticky, yellow coating, and her pulse will be either thready and hesitant or deep and forceful.

Treatment

- To nourish your recipient's Blood and promote her Fluids, use the points BL17, BL20, BL38 and ST36.
- To remove her Heat, use KID6 and SP10.
- To stimulate her Blood flow and specifically affect her bowels, use ST25, because it is a front Mu point.
- To remove stagnation in her bowels, use TW6.

Figure 8.3 The points used for treating constipation.

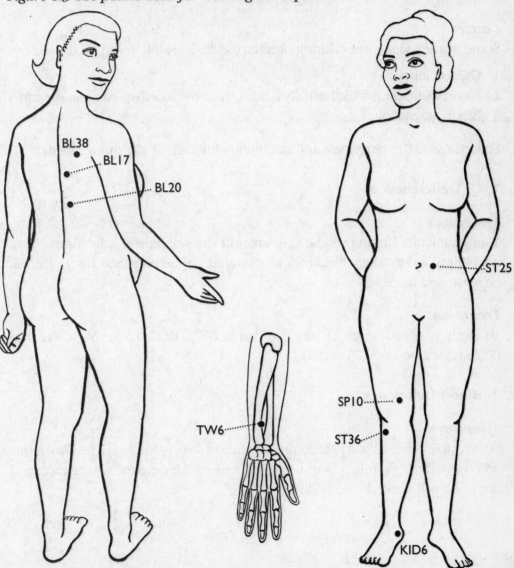

Fainting

Causes
Some women faint either during or after the birth. Fainting can be caused by

1 Qi Deficiency
2 Blood Deficiency, which usually results from haemorrhage during the birth
3 Blood Stagnation.

Following are the symptoms and treatments for each of the three causes.

1 Qi Deficiency

Symptoms
Your recipient's fainting will be sudden, and she will have a pale complexion, cold limbs and a sweaty forehead. Her tongue will be pale, and her pulse will be weak and thready.

Treatment
To tonify your recipient's Qi, use the points BL20, BL22, CV3, CV4, CV12, the GV26 revival point, ST25 and ST36.

2 Blood Deficiency

Symptoms
Your recipient will have a pale complexion and a sweaty forehead, feel nauseous and suffocated, and might have heart palpitations. Her tongue will be pale, and her pulse will be weak and hollow.

Figure 8.4 The points used for treating fainting.

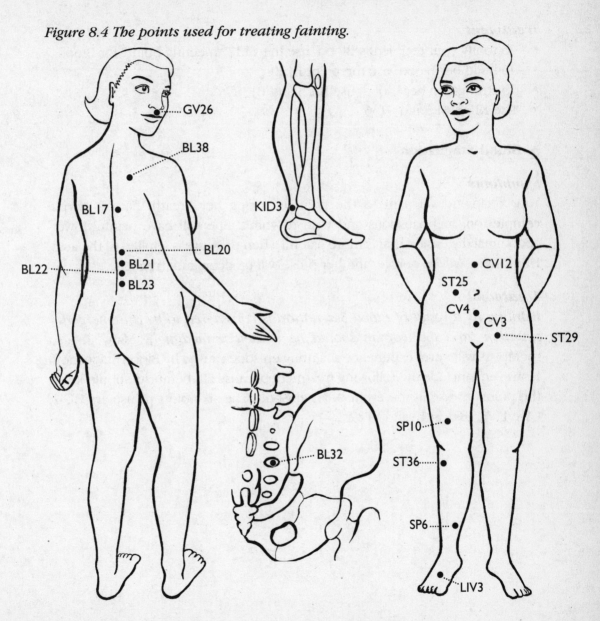

Treatment

- To tonify your recipient's Blood, use the BL17 "meeting point" for Blood.
- To build her Blood, use the point BL20.
- To strengthen her Blood, use BL23 and BL38.
- Use KID3, SP6 and ST36.

3 Blood Stagnation

Symptoms

Your recipient will pant to the point of losing her breath, have a purple complexion, feel nauseous and wish to vomit. She will have painful lower-abdominal distension that is more painful when pressure is applied to the area. Her tongue will be purple, and her pulse will be deep and irregular.

Treatment

Fainting as a result of Blood Stagnation is considered to be an emergency situation, and the woman should be treated immediately. Many Shiatsu therapists will never experience a fainting episode caused by Blood Stagnation. However, I include the following treatment because all therapists should know the points to use in the event of an episode. The six points to use are BL32, CV4, LIV3, SP6, SP10 and ST29.

Insomnia

Causes
Insomnia, or sleeplessness, results from both Heart deficiency and mental stress caused by fatigue experienced during labour. It can be caused by

1 Blood Deficiency
2 Qi Stagnation.

Following are the symptoms and treatments for each of the two causes.

1 Blood Deficiency

Symptoms
Your recipient will be insomniac, have a pale complexion, feel dizzy, have heart palpitations, feel dreamy, wake early, be lethargic and either need or wish to stay in bed. Her tongue will be pale and have a thin coating, and her pulse will be thready and weak.

Treatment
Treatment for insomnia caused by Blood Deficiency involves nourishing your recipient's Qi and Blood, and calming her mind by stroking and caressing her head.

- Sedate the points BL15, BL20, BL23 and HT7.
- Use palming to gently press and rotate your recipient's hypochondrium (the soft area just below the ribs).
- Knead her Hara.
- Sedate KID3, SP6 (gently) and ST36.

2 Qi Stagnation

Symptoms

Your recipient will be insomniac, wake early, be vague, be sad (depressed), sigh, worry and have a feeling of fullness in her chest. Her tongue will be light red and have a thin coating, and her pulse will be stringy.

Treatment

To treat your recipient's insomnia caused by Qi Stagnation, disperse and calm her Liver Qi, nourish her Heart and calm her mind.

- Gently knead your recipient's Hara.
- Sedate the point GV24.
- Pull and sedate HT4 and HT7.
- Apply Jin Shin Do to CV4 and CV6.
- Use your elbows to tonify GB30.
- Sedate KID3 and LIV2.

Figure 8.5 The points used for treating insomnia.

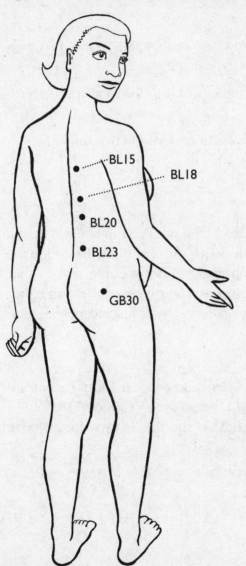
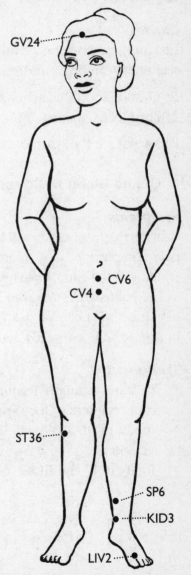

Lactation scantiness

Causes
Lactation, or creation of milk, is aided by Ren Mai Qi and Blood. Lactation scantiness can be caused by

1   Qi and Blood Deficiency as a result of either malnutrition or a strained birth
2   Liver Qi Stagnation.

Following are the symptoms and treatments for each of the two causes.

1 Qi and Blood Deficiency

Symptoms
Your recipient's breasts will be soft and flaccid but not painful. She will have a pale complexion, have blurred vision, be lethargic, feel dizzy, have tinnitus (ringing in the ears), have heart palpitations, have a poor appetite, and feel hot in her palms and soles. Her bowel movements might be irregular, and either her stools will be loose or she will be constipated. Her tongue will be pale, and her pulse will be thready and weak.

Treatment
* Because lactation scantiness is a deficiency issue, you should stimulate your recipient's Qi by applying moxa to the points CV17 and ST18.
* Tonify BL20, ST37 and SI1. The point SI1 is specifically used for affecting lactation.
* Tonify BL17 and BL18.

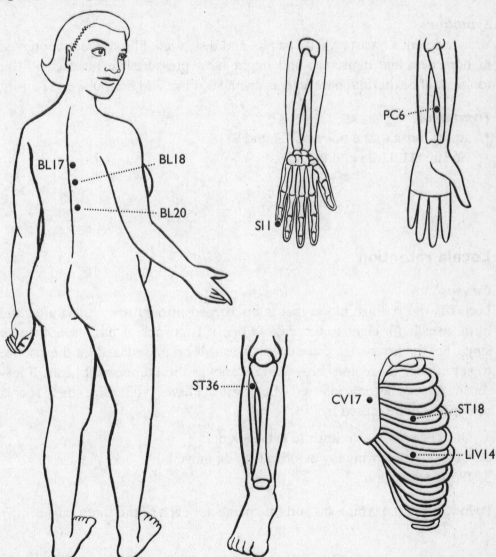

Figure 8.6 The points used for treating lactation scantiness.

2 Liver Qi Stagnation

Symptoms
Your recipient's breasts will be painful and distended. She will feel oppressed in her chest and nauseous, and might have pressure-like headaches. Her tongue will be thin and have a greasy, white coating, and her pulse will be wiry.

Treatment
- Apply moxa to the points CV17 and ST18.
- Sedate SI1, LIV14 and PC6.

Lochia retention

Causes
Lochia is the residual blood that is discharged through the vagina after the birth, usually for eight to ten days. When it is normal, it has an inoffensive smell. For the first two to three days it is usually bright red, and for the last five to seven days it becomes brown and scanty as the uterine wall heals. If it is retained, it can become infected whereby it will have an offensive smell. Lochia retention can be caused by

1 Qi Deficiency, which leads to exhaustion
2 Qi congestion, whereby Blood fails to be moved
3 Blood Stagnation.

Following are the symptoms and treatments for each of the three causes.

1 Qi Deficiency

Symptoms

Your recipient will have a pale, sallow complexion; feel dizzy; have tinnitus (ringing in the ears) and be lethargic; and her lochia discharge will be scanty. Her abdomen might feel empty, and any abdominal distension will be relieved when pressure is applied to the area. Her tongue will be pale and have either minimal or no coating, and her pulse will be fine and weak.

Treatment

- To stimulate your recipient's Qi and Blood, use the points CV4 and CV6.
- To strengthen her in general, use BL17.
- To build her Blood, use BL20.
- To build her Kidney Qi, use BL23.
- To circulate her Qi and Blood, use SP6.
- To facilitate her Qi and Blood flow, use ST36.

2 Qi congestion, whereby Blood fails to be moved

Symptoms

Your recipient's abdomen will be distended, and pain will radiate from her abdomen to both her lower back and her hips. Her tongue will be light red, and her pulse will be wiry.

Treatment

- To improve your recipient's Qi circulation, use the point CV6.
- To improve her Qi and Blood circulation, use ST25.
- To move her Qi and Blood, use ST36.
- To move the Fluids in her Lower Jiao, use BL22.
- To descend her Qi, use ST37.

3 Blood Stagnation

Symptoms

Your recipient will have either scanty or no lochia discharge. She might either vomit or have indigestion (dyspepsia). Her abdomen will be painful, especially when pressure is applied to it; it will also be distended, and might be lumpy. Her tongue will either be slightly purple or have purple markings, and her pulse will be deep and slow.

Treatment

- To move your recipient's Blood, use the points CV4 and SP10.
- To move her stagnant Blood, use ST29.
- To move her Qi and Blood, use SP6.
- To regulate her Blood and Qi, use LIV3.
- To move the stagnant Blood in her uterus, tonify BL32.

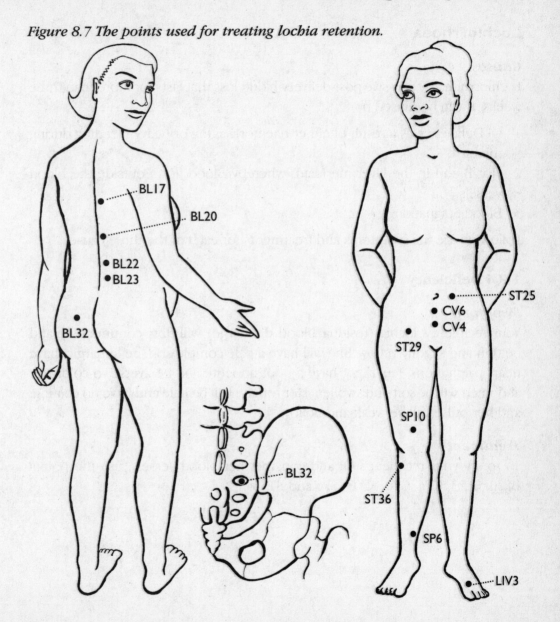

Figure 8.7 The points used for treating lochia retention.

Lochiorrhoea

Causes

Lochiorrhoea is excessive post-delivery blood loss that lasts for more than three weeks. It can be caused by

1 Qi Deficiency, as a result of either haemorrhaging or heavy bleeding during the birth
2 Hot Blood in the Liver meridian, whereby Blood flows outside the blood vessels
3 Blood Stagnation.

Following are the symptoms and treatments for each of the three causes.

1 Qi Deficiency

Symptoms

Your recipient's lochia (residual-blood discharge) will flow continuously, and be thin and slightly yellow. She will have a pale complexion, be lethargic, have heart palpitations, feel dizzy, have a poor appetite and be averse to cold. Her abdomen will be soft and swollen. Her tongue will be pale and have no coating, and her pulse will be weak and hollow.

Treatment

To tonify your recipient's Qi and constrict her blood vessels, use the points BL20, BL23, CV4, CV6, KID3, SP6 and ST36.

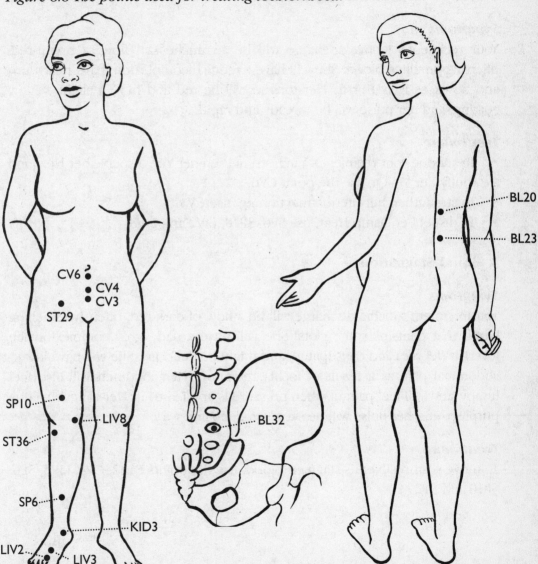

Figure 8.8 The points used for treating lochiorrhoea.

2 Hot Blood in the Liver meridian

Symptoms

Your recipient's lochia discharge will be an unchecked flow of bright-red, offensive-smelling blood. She will have a reddish complexion, have heartburn and be excessively thirsty. Her tongue will be red and have a slight, yellow coating, and her pulse will be thready and rapid.

Treatment

- To subdue your recipient's Yang, strengthen her Yin, disperse her Heat and tonify her Yin Qi, use the point CV6.
- To strengthen her uterine functioning, use CV3.
- To dispel her Damp Heat, use SP6, SP10, LIV2 and LIV8.

3 Blood Stagnation

Symptoms

Your recipient's lochia discharge will be a flow of dark-red, offensive-smelling blood that contains some clots. She will have a dark, grey complexion; be feverish (febrile) and constipated; and might be delirious. She will have lower-abdominal pain as a result of lochia retention. Her abdomen will also feel lumpy, and will feel painful when pressure is applied to it. Her tongue will be purplish, and her pulse will be irregular, deep and wiry.

Treatment

To move your recipient's stagnant Blood, use the points BL32, CV4, LIV3, SP6, SP10 and ST29.

Mastitis

Causes

According to practitioners of Western medicine, mastitis is a breast condition that is usually caused by presence of bacterial infection in either a milk duct or a cracked nipple. Three other causes can be the baby's incorrect suckling, the mother's overindulging in fatty foods and the mother's experiencing emotional disturbances. According to practitioners of Traditional Chinese Medicine, mastitis can also be caused by Qi and Blood Deficiency.

Symptoms

Your recipient's breast area will be both swollen and painful, and either partly or wholly red. She might have either a high temperature or temperature swings. If her condition is caused by Qi and Blood Deficiency, her symptoms will be similar to the ones I have described, and either or both of her breasts will contain hard lumps.

Treatment

- Apply moxa to the points CV17 and ST18.
- To produce a stronger effect, apply moxa to SP8.
- Use BL20, LI11, SP6 and ST36.
- If your recipient's breast is infected, use ST34, which is the specific point for breast infection.
- To affect her Yang Ming, use LI4 and ST18.
- To calm her Internal Wind, use GB20.

Figure 8.9 The points used for treating mastitis.

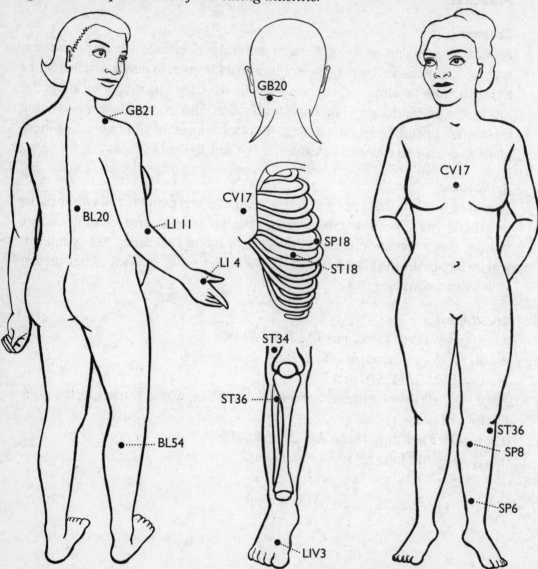

Placenta retention

Causes

Your recipient's placenta might be retained in her body if she is exhausted having had a long and painful birthing. Placenta retention can also be caused by

1   Qi Deficiency
2   Blood Stagnation in the uterus.

The following treatment applies to both causes.

Treatment

To treat placenta retention, strengthen your recipient's Qi and move her Blood.
* To strengthen your recipient's Uterus, use the point CV3.
* To circulate her Qi and Blood, use SP6.
* To help dispel her placenta, use BL60, GB21 and LI4.
* To move her Blood, use CV4 and SP8.
* To move her Qi, use CV6 and SP8; also use ST31, which is the Uterus point.

Figure 8.10 The points used for treating placenta retention.

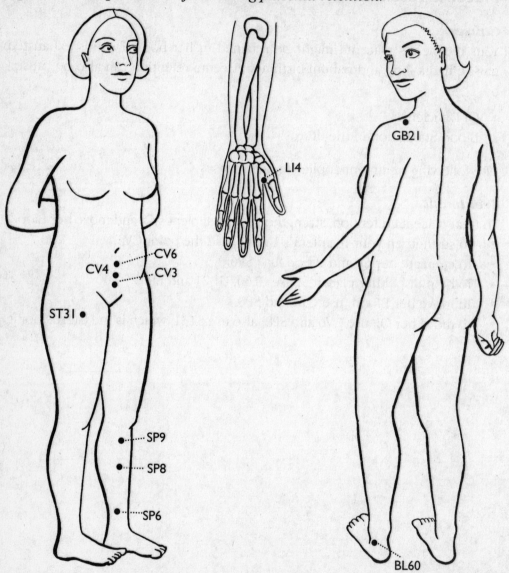

Postnatal depression

Causes

According to practitioners of Traditional Chinese Medicine, postnatal depression is caused by Heart Yin Deficiency as a result of Heart Fire.

Symptoms

Your recipient will be weak in general, be depressed, feel sad, weep, have an unpredictable temper, yawn and sigh frequently, sleep irregularly, be lethargic, have a dry mouth, feel nauseous and be constipated. Her tongue will be red, have minimal coating and have teeth-marked – almost fluted – edges, and her pulse will be weak and stringy, or even thready.

Treatment

- Explain to your postnatally depressed recipient that she will recover more quickly and fully if she undergoes both dietary and herbal therapy. Suggest she undertake dietary adjustments whereby her Spleen, Kidney and Heart meridians will be supported. Suggest she consider avoiding cold, raw foods; alcohol; chilli; curries; fried foods; and greasy foods.
- To support Spleen, suggest she eat all the yellow and orange vegetables. To support Kidney and Heart, suggest that all her food be warm and cooked. Advise her to eat only easily digestible foods. Refer to the section headed "Depression" on pages 83 to 89 of *Chinese Medicine for Women*.
- Treat your postnatally depressed recipient by calming her Liver, strengthening her Spleen, and calming her Heart and Shen.
- Sharply sedate the points BL18, HT9, LI4, PC5 and PC7.
- Gently push and drag your recipient's ribs and firmly press her Hara.
- Sedate the points KID1, LIV2, PC6 and TW5.
- Stroke around her head.
- Support your Shiatsu treatment by sedating LIV3 and SP6.

Figure 8.11 The points used for treating postnatal depression.

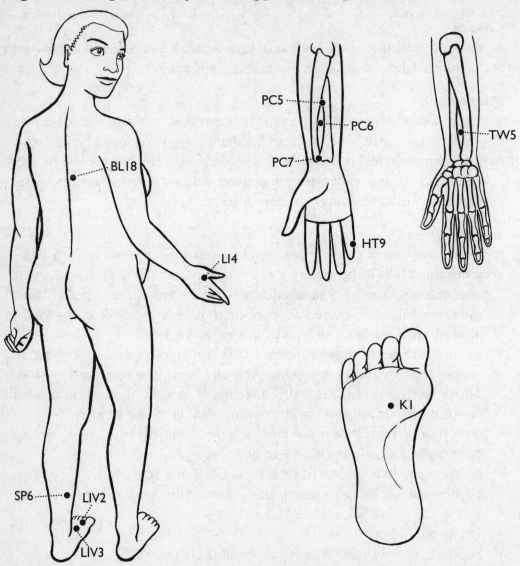

Urinary incontinence

Causes

Urinary incontinence, or inability to control passing of clear urine, can result from the birth. It can be caused by deficiency in general, whereby your recipient's kidneys might be affected. Following are the symptoms and treatment both for when your recipient is deficient in general and when her kidneys are affected.

1 When your recipient is deficient in general

Symptoms

Your recipient will be lethargic, her tongue will be pale and her pulse will be hollow.

Treatment

Use the points CV3, CV4, ST25 and ST36.

2 When your recipient's kidneys are affected

Symptoms

Your recipient will have a slightly dark complexion, and her lower back or knees will either ache or be weak. These symptoms are usually associated with Kidney Deficiency. Her tongue will be very moist, and her pulse will be deep.

Figure 8.12 The points used for treating urinary incontinence.

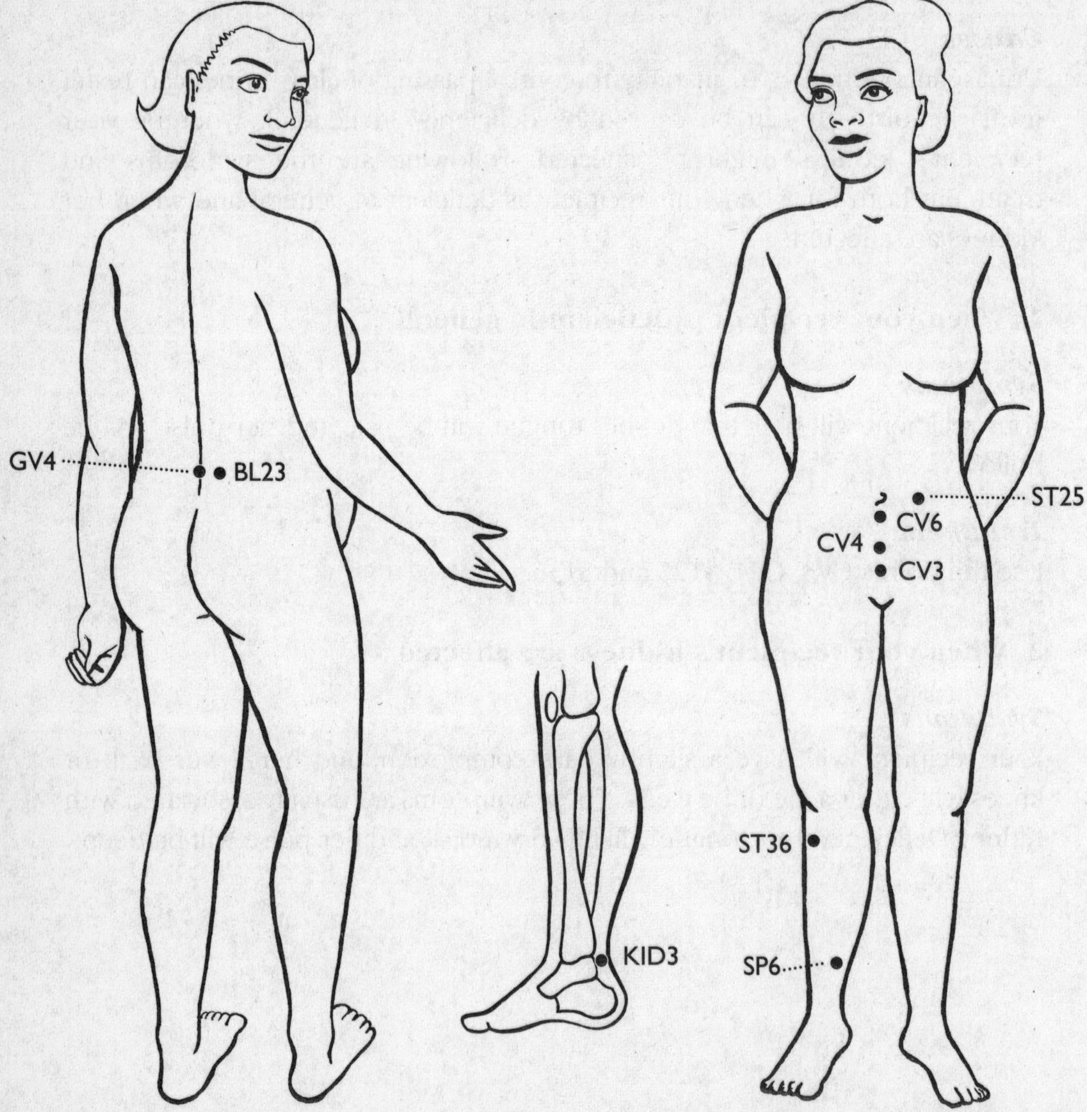

GV4 ········ BL23

ST25

CV6

CV4

CV3

KID3

ST36

SP6

Treatment

Instruct your recipient to exercise her pelvic-floor muscles: to squeeze and relax her anal muscles then squeeze and relax her vaginal muscles (see page 176 of "Chapter 10: Exercise therapy" and Figure 10.1 on page 177). Recommend she do the exercise as often as possible, both day and night, until she regains some control of her pelvic-floor muscles.

- Use the Shiatsu points for deficiency in general: CV3, CV4, ST25 and ST36.
- Apply moxa to GV4.
- Use BL23, KID3 and SP6.

9
Lifestyle and dietary therapy

Lifestyle therapy

Lifestyle is a difficult area for Shiatsu therapists to counsel their recipients about. We wish our recipients to reduce their stress and thereby calm their Liver Qi and enable their Shen to reside in the Heart. Because of our recipients' modern-day environment and life situation, it can be almost impossible for us to effectively reduce their stress.

You should balance your lifestyle suggestions with providing an effective Shiatsu treatment. When you are treating your recipient, always give her emotional support and strength.

Reducing stress

I try to make my pregnant Shiatsu recipients aware of how stress, diet and drugs affect both their body and their mind. My intention is to raise their awareness about the harm they might be doing themselves. I encourage them to elevate their feet, to get plenty of rest and to nap regularly if possible. I tell them it is appropriate to try and reduce their workload, any demanding exercise regimen and any emotional or physical stress.

Undergoing Shiatsu therapy on a regular basis can help counteract the effects of any stressors. The therapist should consider stress reduction both with reference to each recipient's needs and within the confines of each recipient's situation.

When you are counselling the pregnant woman about the effects of her lifestyle, be aware that she might have to work for as long as possible up to her estimated date of delivery (EDD), for financial and/or personal reasons.

Dietary therapy
Following are some dietary suggestions for you to make to your Shiatsu recipient.

Types of food
Help your pregnant recipient strengthen her Qi and Blood by suggesting that as much as possible she ingest well-cooked, easily digestible, warm foods and drinks.

Creating an eating plan
Suggest your recipient create an eating plan in which she includes food that both supports Spleen and Kidney and regulates Liver Qi.

Meal sizes
Suggest your recipient eat a large breakfast, a medium-size lunch and a smallish dinner.

Coffee
Explain to your recipient that she should try to eliminate coffee from her diet because it constricts blood flow.

Alcohol
Explain to your recipient that she should avoid alcohol because it causes over-heating in the body.

Fatty foods
Explain to your recipient that she should avoid fatty foods because they dampen Spleen Qi.

Kelp
If your recipient eats kelp, explain that she should reduce her intake of it because it contains a lot of salt.

Recreational drugs
Explain to your recipient that she should avoid taking recreational drugs because they deplete Kidney Qi.

The dietary regimen
Always consider your recipient's current dietary regimen. If she cannot incorporate Japanese, Chinese or macrobiotic foods in her diet because they are not to her taste, help her consider alternative menu choices she can realistically incorporate in her menus.

Spleen, Liver and Heart
Explain that when a woman is pregnant, it is necessary for her Spleen to be strengthened and for her Liver and Heart to be calmed. Always help your recipient consider foods that meet these needs: reduce – or better still eliminate altogether – raw, cold foods, and replace them with cooked, warm foods.

Morning sickness

The two most common causes of morning sickness are

1 imbalance as a result of rising Liver Yang
2 imbalance as a result of Spleen Qi Deficiency.

Increased Yang or activity

Explain to your recipient that because the foetus is growing rapidly, she will be more Yang and her body temperature will consequently increase.

Individual pregnant women's diet

Be aware it is not possible to recommend a specific diet for any pregnant Shiatsu recipient because her diet style will be affected by her individual characteristics, environment and tastes. You can, however, suggest she consider the following dietary guidelines when she is making her decisions about what to eat.

Some dietary guidelines for the pregnant woman to consider

1 Try to eat seasonal fruit and vegetables, and eat them at the temperature that is appropriate for the season; for example, eat warm foods in winter.
2 Prefer locally grown foods.
3 Make sure at least 50 per cent of your diet consists of grains and carbo-hydrates.
4 Make sure at least 30 per cent of your diet consists of vegetables.
5 If you eat meat, it can constitute between 10 and 20 per cent of your diet. Eat mainly chicken and fish, and reduce the amount of red meat you eat.
6 Reduce processed and preserved foods. It is advisable to reduce the amount of soft cheeses and sliced meat you eat, because of the possible activity of Listeria bacteria, which can affect the health of the embryo and foetus.
7 Reduce your intake of greasy, fatty foods.

8 Do not eat nuts very often: they have a high fat content and can be difficult to digest.

9 Reduce your intake of coffee; teas; alcohol; and sweet, cold, fizzy drinks.

10 To support your Spleen and Stomach functions, chew your food well, until it is liquefied in your mouth.

11 Whenever you eat, be seated, comfortable and peaceful.

12 When you have finished eating, leave the table satisfied, not full.

13 When you are thirsty, drink warm water.

14 Do not eat for up to three hours before you go to bed. Eating within three hours of bed time can cause either Spleen Qi Stagnation or food stagnation in the intestines.

15 Engage in mild activity such as walking, yoga or Tai Chi.

16 Cook your food using either gas or slow electric heating, not a microwave oven. Reserve your microwave for heating food that has already been cooked either in a conventional oven or on the stovetop.

Soups

Soups are one of the easiest foods to both make and digest. Many of my pregnant Shiatsu recipients have readily incorporated a hearty soup in their breakfast. Soups for the pregnant woman should contain either barley or rice in order to reduce oedema (fluid build-up and retention). Soups made with bones and vegetables are another excellent choice. This is because the bones help strengthen Blood, the vegetables contribute fibre, and the soup has to be served warm in order to both be palatable and support Spleen.

Porridge

Porridge is a good choice for the pregnant woman if she cannot either incorporate rice in her soups or make rice porridge (congee). Porridge is sometimes not suggested in any treatment for Spleen Qi Deficiency. However, it is a good source of carbohydrates and a source of sustained energy whereby the pregnant woman can make it to lunchtime without having to resort to sugar-type energy boosters. In my Shiatsu practice, eating porridge has not had any dampening effects on Damp recipients; in fact, it seems to support movement of Damp.

Juices
If your recipient enjoys drinking fruit juices and, say, carrot juice, suggest she dilute them with 50 per cent water and drink them as warm as possible.

Cravings during pregnancy
Experiencing cravings is a normal part of any woman's pregnancy. Cravings are caused by sudden changes that occur in Yin and Yang whereby Spleen and Stomach are affected. The cravings can be viewed as being the body's way of trying to create balance. For the pregnant woman, it is better to try and satisfy rather than attempt to suppress them.

Sometimes it is possible to substitute a "healthy" food for a food that is craved, and following are some suggestions.

Craving oily or fatty foods
If your recipient is craving oily or fatty foods, suggest she eat either sautéed vegetables or fried rice. She might also be satisfied by eating popped corn served with a small amount of sesame oil, not butter.

Craving sweet foods
If your recipient is craving sweet foods, suggest she eat cooked fruit as well as sweet vegetables such as carrot, pumpkin and swede.

Craving sour foods
If your recipient is craving sour foods, suggest she eat umeboshi plums.

Craving fruit

If your recipient is craving tropical and/or raw fruit, suggest she eat cooked fruit and include dry fruits with it.

Some suggestions for relieving five common pregnancy-related problems

1 To relieve morning sickness

- Before you rise in the morning, prepare a tea using fresh-apple peel and rice. To make the tea, mix between 30 and 60 grams of fresh-apple peel and 30 grams of rice that has been fried until it is yellowish.
- Prepare a tea using between 15 and 20 grams of grapefruit peel boiled in water.
- Prepare ginger tea, preferably using fresh ginger.
- To relieve nausea, suck umeboshi-plum pulp and eat the plums' skin. Whether or not you try this remedy will depend on your personal taste preferences.

2 To increase lactation

- Prepare a soup using 10 grams of anise seeds and a small amount of wine.
- Prepare a soup using 150 grams of soya-bean curd, 50 grams of brown rice and three cups of water.
- Prepare a chicken-and-rice soup.
- Prepare a pea-and-ham soup. Eating this soup also helps build Blood.

3 To treat mastitis

For acute mastitis the onset of which is within two or three days of the birth, drink one cup of the following mixture in the morning and one cup in the evening. Add 40 grams of dry mandarin peel and 7 grams of licorice root to two cups of water. Bring the mixture to the boil, then cool it and boil it again. Drink the mixture warm.

4 *To treat Cold Invasion after the birth*

Add 5 grams of powdered cinnamon to one cup of rice wine. Drink the mixture three times a day.

5 *To treat constipation during pregnancy*

* Both in the morning and at night, eat one tablespoon of the following creamy mixture. Combine 15 grams of sweet-apricot seeds and 30 grams each of rice and sugar. Add some water, crush the three ingredients and mix them to a creamy consistency.
* To help lubricate the bowels, drink a tablespoon of honey mixed with a glass of warm water every morning.

10
Exercise therapy

If the pregnant Shiatsu recipient is able to exercise, the therapist should advise her to undertake gentle exercise on a regular basis. The therapist should inform his or her recipient about the following three main benefits of exercising during pregnancy.

The three main benefits of exercise during pregnancy

1 It both strengthens the muscles that support the internal organs and improves Blood and Qi circulation in the pelvic cavity.
2 It improves the respiratory and circulatory functions that support the metabolic process.
3 When the woman breathes correctly while she is exercising on a regular basis, her diaphragm and abdominal muscles are being strengthened, and her labour and recovery will thereby be facilitated.

Relieving lower-back ache

Lower-back ache is a major issue for most women throughout their whole pregnancy. It can be temporarily relieved by applying localised heat to the area in the form of either a small bag of dry wheat heated in the microwave or a hot-water bottle. Hot-water bottles should not be left to cool too much; if they are, the lower-back area can be subject to Cold Invasion.

The pelvic-floor muscles

Pregnancy and labour can weaken both the pelvic-floor muscles and the abdominal wall. The pelvic-floor muscles form a "figure 8" around the vagina and anus, as shown in Figure 10.1. This weakening can then cause the uterus, vagina and other internal organs to prolapse, and the prolapsing in turn can cause bowel and/or bladder (urinary) incontinence.

The pelvic-floor exercise

I have already described the pelvic-floor exercise in the section headed "Urinary incontinence" in "Chapter 8: Conditions that might occur after the birth". This simple exercise can be undertaken both during pregnancy and after the birth; at any time and as often as possible; and while the woman is sitting, standing or walking.

Most women find it easiest to sit when they are doing the exercise for the first time. All that is required is to tighten then relax the anal and vaginal sphincter muscles, one after the other, in sequence. You breathe in while you are tightening your anal sphincter muscle, hold for a count of five, then relax the muscle while you are breathing out. You then repeat the exercise using your vaginal muscle.

Figure 10.1 The female external genitalia and the "figure 8" formed by the pelvic-floor muscles.

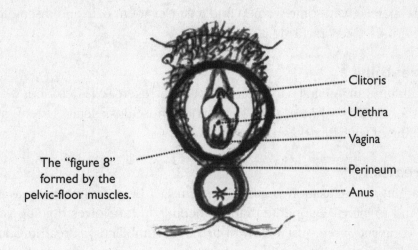

The "figure 8" formed by the pelvic-floor muscles.

Clitoris

Urethra

Vagina

Perineum

Anus

Gentle exercise

To aid Spleen Qi movement, the pregnant woman could undertake a gentle, fifteen-minute walk every day. Gentle stretching in the form of yoga is also beneficial during pregnancy.

If the woman has had a normal birth, she can undertake gentle exercise between twelve and sixteen hours afterwards in order to restore the strength and muscle tone of her pelvic and abdominal muscles. Gentle exercise both helps the uterus return to its normal shape more quickly and aids the functioning of the bowels. However, the woman should exercise slowly and gently, because if she exercises too vigorously, her Spleen's holding ability will be damaged and cause prolapse of the uterus, or worse.

Tai Chi

Tai Chi is of great benefit if the woman has been practising it before she became pregnant; however, practising it can be difficult if she starts after she becomes pregnant, especially during the third trimester. Because it involves moving in a slow and restrained way, some women find it causes them pain and discomfort if they are not used to practising it.

Deep breathing

Deep breathing is an integral part of all the following exercises I describe. When you breathe deeply, you support both your musculoskeletal system and strengthening of your Blood and Qi.

Hara breathing

Hara breathing, or relaxation breathing, seems to help reduce nausea and vomiting and to increase appetite that has been lost. It involves holding your palms to your abdomen, just below your navel (umbilicus). Breathing in a relaxed way, you relax and let all your thoughts and awareness go to the area you are resting your palms on. You remain aware of the rising and falling of your abdomen but do not concentrate too hard on your abdominal area. After a while, you might notice that your abdomen is gently rising and falling with each breath you take.[15]

When not to exercise

It is not appropriate to exercise either during pregnancy or after the birth if any of the following five conditions are present.

1 Acute inflammation of the reproductive organs
2 High fever
3 A pelvic abscess

4 A tumour

5 Excessive bleeding

If the woman has a history of habitual miscarriage, she should not exercise during the first trimester.

Nine pregnancy exercises

I recommend that the pregnant woman commence the following nine exercises between the fourth and six months of pregnancy. If you are a Shiatsu therapist, you should remind your recipient to undertake all the movements slowly and softly and that she should not feel fatigued after undertaking them.

Exercise 1

- This exercise is for restoring Qi to your hands and feet after you have been asleep and for supporting Liver Qi's smooth flowing of Qi function. It is best to undertake the exercise in bed, when you have just woken up.
- Lie on your back, stretch your legs out, and place your arms by your side. Grasp and scratch your hands and feet fifty times, then relax. See Figure 10.2.

Figure 10.2   Exercise 1: for restoring Qi.

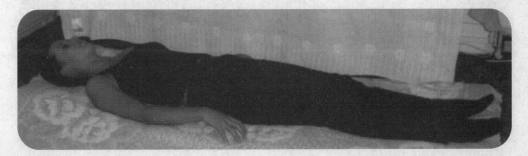

Exercise 2

- This exercise is for supporting smooth flowing of Qi, Blood and Fluids to your extremities (hands and feet).
- Lie on your back, relax and extend your legs, and place your arms by your side. Roll your arms inwards then outwards fifty times. Roll your legs inwards then outwards fifty times. See Figure 10.3.

Figure 10.3   Exercise 2: for toning the extremities.

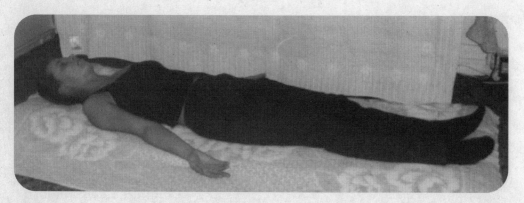

Exercise 3

- This exercise is for helping stretch your perineum and for strengthening your pelvic-floor muscles.
- Lie on your back, and keep your legs straight and together. Bend your knees, and draw your heels up to your buttocks. Lift your pelvis as you tighten your anal muscle, then lower your pelvis as you relax your anal muscle. Keep your hips down, face your soles together, and let your legs drop down. Breathe in and out deeply three times. Extend your legs and relax. Do the exercise ten times. See Figure 10.4.

Figure 10.4   Exercise 3: for stretching the perineum.

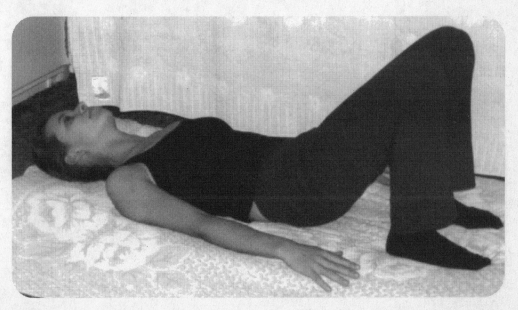

Exercise 4

- This exercise is for releasing tension in your shoulders and arms.
- Lie on your back, stretch your arms out, and keep your legs together. Imagine you are lying in the shape of a cross (+). See Figure 10.5a. Keep your hips as still as possible, and extend your right hand across your body to your left arm. Then extend your left hand across your body to your right arm, and rest. See Figure 10.5b. Do the exercise ten times.

Figure 10.5a   Exercise 4: lying in the shape of a cross.

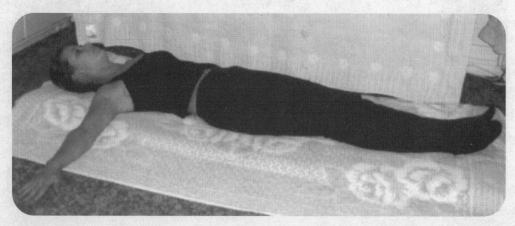

Figure 10.5b   Exercise 4: for releasing tension.

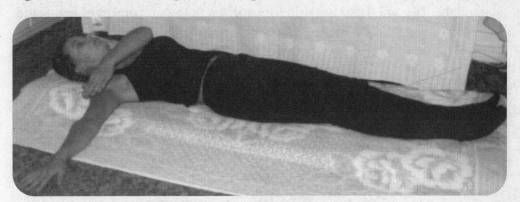

Exercise 5

- This is the pelvic-floor exercise, for helping treat urinary (bladder) incontinence and strengthening your pelvic-floor muscles.
- Lie on your back, and relax your arms and legs. Inhale, and tense your anal sphincter muscle; then exhale, and relax the muscle. Do this first part of the exercise between twenty and thirty times. Inhale, and tense your vaginal sphincter muscle; then exhale, and relax the muscle. Do this second part of the exercise between twenty and thirty times.

Exercise 6

- This exercise is for releasing some of the tension that builds up in your hips and for stretching your Bladder meridian. I suggest you incorporate it in your exercise regimen slowly, because it might be too vigorous to start off with.
- Stand, and place your hands on your hips. Leading with your left leg, take a long step forward. Do not take too big a step, otherwise you will overbalance.

Your front leg should be bent, your back leg straight. Then stand up straight. Take another long step forward, leading with your right leg. Stand up straight again. Do the exercise six times. See Figure 10.6.

Figure 10.6   Exercise 6: for stretching the hips.

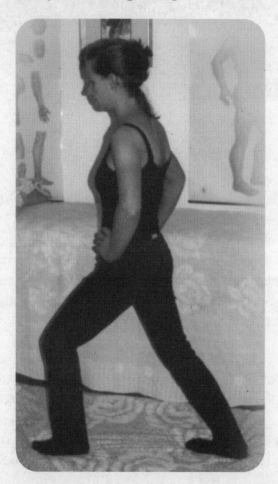

Exercise 7

- This exercise is for helping strengthen your lower legs and relieving your hips.
- Stand, and place your hand on your hips. Do not bend your knees, and lift your left heel off the ground. Do this first part of the exercise six times. Then, again keeping your legs straight, lift your right heel off the ground. Do this second part of the exercise six times. See Figure 10.7.

Figure 10.7   Exercise 7: for releasing the legs.

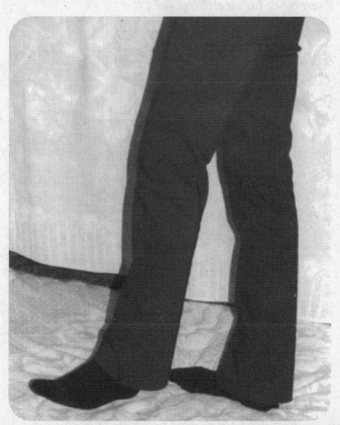

Exercise 8

- This exercise is for stretching your hips.
- Stand, place your hands on your hips, and lift your left knee as high as possible. Do not lean forward, and lift your knee only as high as is comfortable. You might have to use a chair for support. Do this first part of the exercise six times. Then lift your right knee as high as possible six times. See Figure 10.8.

Figure 10.8   Exercise 8: for stretching the hips.

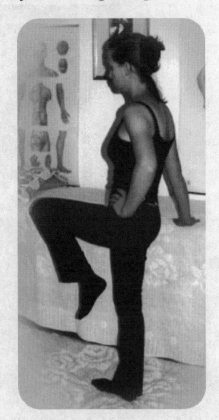

Exercise 9

- This is a good exercise with which to finish your exercise regimen, because it is a gentle cooling-off exercise and relieves your ankles. Alternatively, it can be used as a good warm-up exercise for your regimen.
- Stand, and place your hands on your hips. Rotate your left ankle from left to right then right to left. Do this first part of the exercise six times. Then rotate your right ankle from left to right then right to left six times.

Specific exercises for four conditions that might occur during pregnancy

Try gentle exercises 10, 11, 12 or 13 if you wish to relieve nausea, help stretch your perineum, treat constipation or relieve oedema. Make sure you get plenty of rest as well as exercise during your pregnancy. When you rest, always incorporate elevation of your legs in order to ease oedema and support flowing of venous blood. When you get plenty of rest, your Heart Blood is also able to rest and your Shen is supported in being housed in your Heart.

Exercise 10: For relieving nausea

- This is the Hara-breathing exercise, or relaxation-breathing exercise, for relieving nausea and vomiting and for increasing appetite that has been lost.
- Hold your palms to your abdomen, just below your navel (umbilicus). Breathe in a relaxed way, relax, and let all your thoughts and awareness go to the area you are resting your palms on. Remain aware of the rising and falling of your abdomen, but do not concentrate too hard on your abdominal area. After a while, notice that your abdomen is gently rising and falling with each breath you take. See Figure 10.9 on page 188.

Figure 10.9   Exercise 10: for relieving nausea.

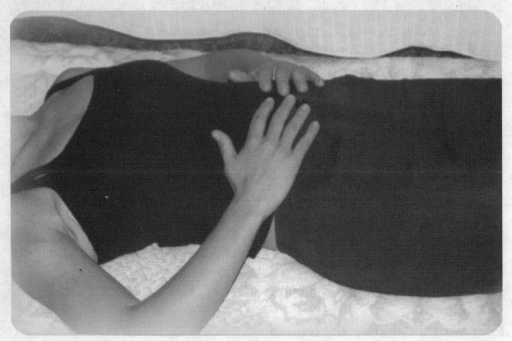

Exercise 11: For helping stretch the perineum

- This exercise is for strengthening your abdominal, pelvic and inner-thigh muscles and relaxing your lower back.
- Lie on your back, bend your knees, face your soles together, and drop your knees open to the side. Draw your bent legs as close to your body as is comfortable, and place your arms by your sides. Inhale deeply. Exhale, and tighten your abdominal muscles so your tummy is flattened and so your spine is lengthened and flattened to the floor. Press your heels together, and let your knees move towards each other slightly. You should feel the

stretch in your inner thighs. Inhale, relax your hips, and let your knees drop open. Do the exercise six times a day. See Figure 10.4 on page 181.

Exercise 12: For treating constipation

Squat by bending your knees and keeping your buttocks lower than your knees. Try to tighten then relax your anal sphincter muscle. Do the exercise twice a day until you have regular bowel movements. See Figure 10.10.

Figure 10.10   Exercise 12: for treating constipation.

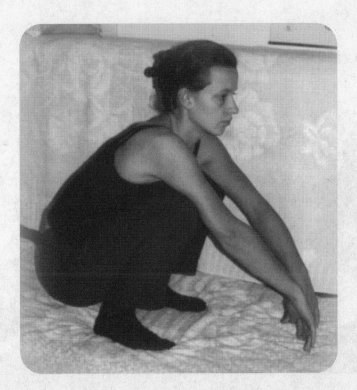

Exercise 13: For relieving oedema

Lie on your back, place your arms by your sides, bend your legs, and point your feet to the wall. Keep your heels on the wall, and raise your legs. Hold the position for one to two minutes, then return to your starting position. Do the exercise between three and five times. See Figure 10.11.

Figure 10.11   Exercise 13: for relieving oedema.

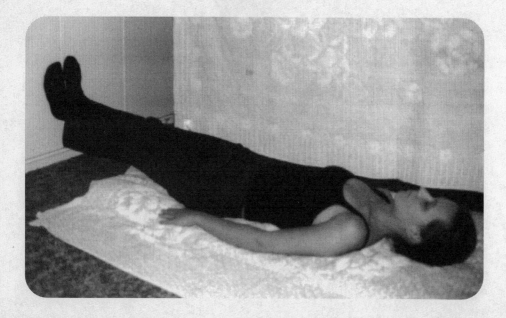

Specific exercises for seven conditions that might occur after the birth

Exercises 14–20 supplement the new mother's recovery. During labour, the woman's abdominal and pelvic-floor muscles are worked hard, and these seven exercises can help return the muscles to close to their original condition. The exercises also help move both Qi and Blood.

When not to undertake the seven exercises

If you are a new mother who
- has given birth by caesarian section,
- has a high fever,
- is bleeding heavily, or
- has lost a lot of blood during the birth,

you should postpone undertaking these exercises until you have fully recovered.

The exercises

If your birthing was normal, you should be able to commence the exercises within twenty-four hours.
- Choose only *two or three* of the seven exercises to continue with.
- Do only as many repetitions as you feel comfortable with, and *stop if you have any pain*.
- Let your body determine how far you take your exercise regimen: there is no hard-and-fast rule.
- Remember that you might not be able to exercise as you did before you were pregnant, and remember to gradually increase your level of exercise to what it was formerly.

Hara breathing

You will facilitate your recovery if you practise Hara breathing from the first day after your birthing. Hara breathing calms your Shen and promotes good blood flow through your pelvic cavity.

Eight instructions to follow

1   When you are doing the exercises, concentrate on performing a lifting action internally. Do not push outwards, otherwise you will damage either your internal organs or your Spleen Qi and Kidney Qi.

2   Exercises 14, 15 and 16 can usually be undertaken twenty-four hours after the birth.

3   Exercises 14, 15, 16 and 17 can be undertaken from the third day after the birth.

4   Exercises 14, 15, 16, 17, 18 and 19 can be undertaken from the fourth day after the birth.

5   All seven exercises can be undertaken from the sixth day after the birth.

6   For the first five days after the birth, do the exercises five times each.

7   From the sixth day after the birth, do the exercises twelve times each.

8   Do the exercises in sequence.

Exercise 14

Lie on your back, and place your arms by your sides. Inhale, and lift your arms up. Exhale, and slowly lower your arms. If you feel strain in your lower back, reduce the strain by bending your knees and resting your feet on the floor. See Figure 10.12.

Figure 10.12   Exercise 14.

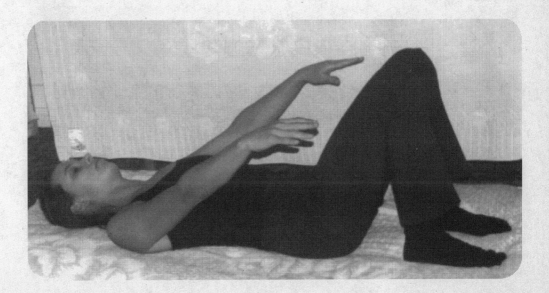

Exercise 15

Lie on your back, and bend your knees. Inhale, and gently raise your left leg. Exhale, and lower the leg. Inhale, and gently raise your right leg. Exhale, and lower the leg. See Figure 10.13.

Figure 10.13   Exercise 15.

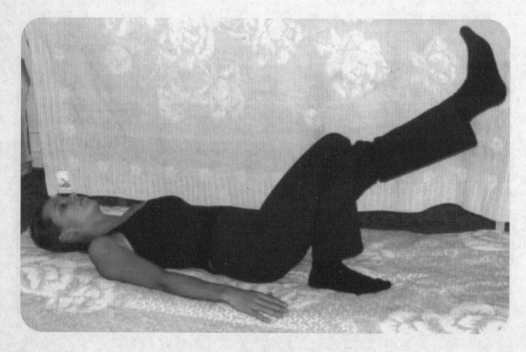

Exercise 16

Lie on your back, and bend your knees. Inhale, and lift your bent legs from your hips as far as is comfortable. Exhale, and lower your legs. See Figure 10.14.

Figure 10.14   Exercise 16.

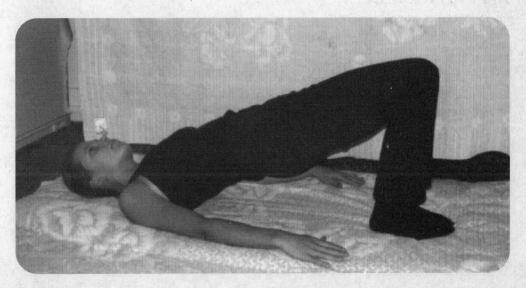

Exercise 17

Lie on your left side, relax your legs, and rest your right leg on your left leg. Inhale, and lift your *right* leg, scissor-like, to a comfortable height. Exhale, and lower the leg. Lie on your right side, relax your legs, and rest your left leg on your right leg. Inhale, and lift your *left* leg, scissor-like, to a comfortable height. Exhale, and lower the leg. See Figure 10.15.

Figure 10.15   Exercise 17.

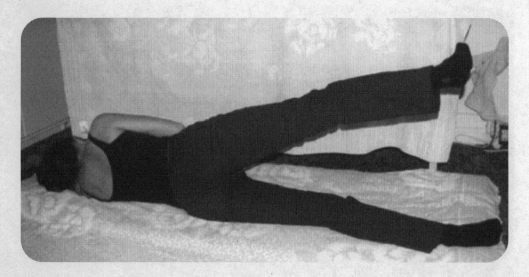

Exercise 18

Lie on your stomach, and bend your knees. Press your heels together as close as possible to your buttocks. Exhale, and lower your legs to be straight again. See Figure 10.16.

Figure 10.16   Exercise 18.

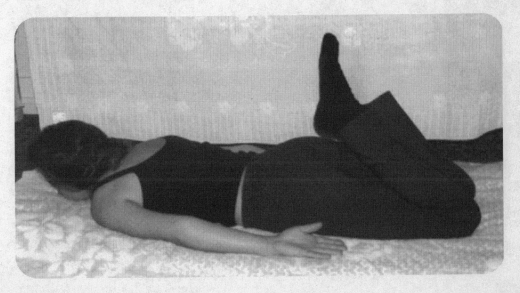

Exercise 19

Lie on your back, and bend your knees. Do slow sit-ups, and come up only as far as is comfortable. Use your arms for support while you are doing the sit-ups. See Figure 10.17. When your strength returns, do the exercise without using your arms for support.

Figure 10.17   Exercise 19.

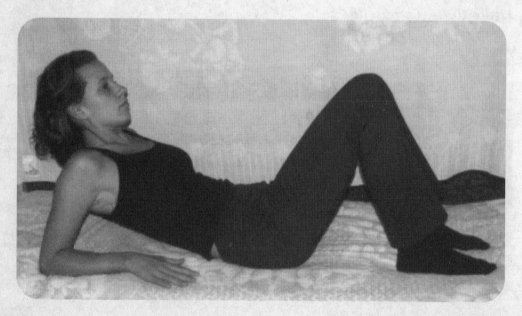

Exercise 20

Lie on your back, and stretch your arms out for balance. Move your legs as if you were pedalling a bicycle. See Figure 10.18. Alternatively, use your arms for supporting your hips if your hips require more support. Breathe slowly and regularly while you are pedalling.

Figure 10.18   Exercise 20.

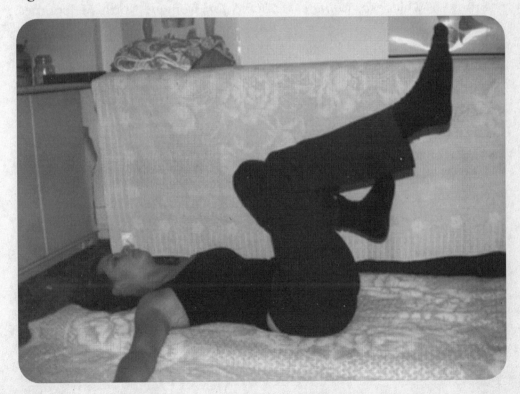

Endnotes

[1] Bronwyn Whitlocke, *Chinese Medicine for Women*, North Melbourne: Spinifex Press, 1997, page 20.

[2] Bronwyn Whitlocke, *Chinese Medicine for Women*, North Melbourne: Spinifex Press, 1997, page 21.

[3] Bronwyn Whitlocke, *Chinese Medicine for Women*, North Melbourne: Spinifex Press, 1997, page 6.

[4] Bronwyn Whitlocke, *Chinese Medicine for Women*, North Melbourne: Spinifex Press, 1997, page 3.

[5] Bronwyn Whitlocke, *Chinese Medicine for Women*, North Melbourne: Spinifex Press, 1997, page 21.

[6] Bronwyn Whitlocke, *Chinese Medicine for Women*, North Melbourne: Spinifex Press, 1997, page 21.

[7] Endo Ryokyo, *Tao Shiatsu*, New York: Japan Publications, 1995, page 80.

[8] Giovanni Maciocia, *The Foundations of Chinese Medicine*, New York: Churchill Livingstone, 1989, page 4.

[9] Wataru Ohashi and Mary M. Hoover, *Natural Childbirth, the Eastern Way*, New York: Ballantine Books, 1983, page 19.

[10] Giovanni Maciocia, *The Foundations of Chinese Medicine*, New York: Churchill Livingstone, 1989, page 37.

[11] Giovanni Maciocia, *The Foundations of Chinese Medicine*, New York: Churchill Livingstone, 1989, page 38.

[12] Li Shi Zhen, *Pulse Diagnosis*, Massachusetts: Paradigm Press, 1981, page 22.

[13] Endo Ryokyo, *Tao Shiatsu*, New York: Japan Publications, 1995, page 76.

[14] *Cathay Herbs Newsletter*, Summer 1996 issue, Sydney: Cathay Herbs, page 2.

[15] Bronwyn Whitlocke, *Chinese Medicine for Women*, North Melbourne: Spinifex Press, 1997, page 47.

References

Chang, Edward C. *Knocking at the Gate of Life*. Pennsylvania: Rodale Press, 1985.

Fream, William C. *Notes on Obstetrics*. New York: Churchill Livingstone, 1982.

Ghangying, Tian. *Chinese Massage Therapy*. People's Republic of China: Shandong Science and Technology Press, 1990.

Kushi, Michio and Aveline. *Macrobiotic Pregnancy and Care of the Newborn*. New York: Japan Publications, 1984.

Leeguarden, Iona M. *Acupressure Way of Health*. New York: Japan Publications, 1990.

Liang, Zhang Ting. *A Handbook of Traditional Chinese Medicine*. Beijing: Shandong Science and Technology Press, 1991.

Llewellyn-Jones, Derek. *Fundamentals of Obstetrics and Gynaecology*. London: Faber & Faber, 1966.

Lowe, Royston. *Acupuncture in Gynaecology and Obstetrics*. Northamptonshire: Thorsons Publishing Group, 1990.

Maciocia, Giovanni. *Tongue Diagnosis in Chinese Medicine*. Seattle: Eastland Press, 1987.

Masunaga, Shizuto and Ohashi, Wataru. *Zen Shiatsu*. New York: Japan Publications, 1988.

Namikoshi, Toru. *Complete Book of Shiatsu Therapy*. New York: Japan Publications, 1989.

Ohashi, Wataru. *Do It Yourself Shiatsu*. London: Mandala Books (Unwin Publishing), 1977.

Ohashi, Wataru and Hoover, Mary M. *Natural Childbirth, the Eastern Way*. New York: Ballantine Books, 1983.

Reed Gach, Michael. *AcuYoga*. New York: Japan Publications, 1981.

Ryokyo, Endo. *Tao Shiatsu*. New York: Japan Publications, 1995.

References

Sinclair, C. C. R. and Webb, J. B. *Aids to Undergraduate Obstetrics and Gynaecology*. New York: Churchill Livingstone, 1986.

Varma, Thankham R. *Manual of Gynaecology*. New York: Churchill Livingstone, 1986.

Whitlocke, Bronwyn. *Chinese Medicine for Women*. North Melbourne: Spinifex Press, 1997.

Zhen, Li Shi. *Pulse Diagnosis*. Massachusetts: Paradigm Press, 1981.

Zhou, Dahong. *Chinese Exercise Book*. Australia and New Zealand: Sacred Black Row Press, 1984.

Index

If you would like to know more about Spinifex Press,
write for a free catalogue or visit our Home Page.

SPINIFEX PRESS

PO Box 212, North Melbourne, Victoria 3051, Australia

http://www.spinifexpress.com.au